THE PUBLIC HEALTH
RESEARCHER

THE PUBLIC HEALTH
RESEARCHER

A METHODOLOGICAL GUIDE

JEANNE DALY

ALLAN KELLEHEAR

MICHAEL GLIKSMAN

Melbourne

OXFORD UNIVERSITY PRESS

Oxford Auckland New York

OXFORD UNIVERSITY PRESS AUSTRALIA

Oxford   New York
Athens   Auckland   Bangkok   Bombay
Calcutta   Cape Town   Dar es Salaam   Delhi
Florence   Hong Kong   Istanbul   Karachi
Kuala Lumpur   Madras   Madrid   Melbourne
Mexico City   Nairobi   Paris   Port Moresby
Singapore   Taipei   Tokyo   Toronto

and associated companies in
Berlin   Ibadan

OXFORD is a trade mark of Oxford University Press

National Library of Australia
Cataloguing-in-Publication data:

Daly, J. M. (Jeanne Marguerite), 1940– .
   The public health researcher: a methodological guide.

   Bibliography.
   Includes index.
   ISBN 0 19 554075 1.

   1. Public health — Research. 2. Public health — Research
   — Methodology. I. Kellehear, Allan. II. Gliksman, Michael
   David. III. Title.

362.1072

Edited by Lucy Davison
Indexed by Max McMaster
Text design by Steve Randles
Cover design and illustrations by Anitra Blackford
Typeset by Desktop Concepts P/L, Melbourne
Printed through Bookpac Production Services, Singapore
Published by Oxford University Press,
253 Normanby Road, South Melbourne, Australia

Contents

Abbreviations

AIDS	acquired immune deficiency syndrome
CO	carbon monoxide
Hib	haemophilus influenzae type b
HIV	human immunodeficiency virus
HRT	hormone replacement therapy
MAL	meta-analysis of literature
MAP	meta-analysis of individual patient data
QALY	quality-adjusted life year
RCT	randomised control trial
SAQ	self-assessment questionnaire
SLE	systemic lupus erythematosus
SMR	Standardised Mortality Ratio

Preface

What methods does the present-day public health researcher need to know? Once upon a time, and not too long ago either, the answer to that question might have been simply 'epidemiological methods' — that is, surveys, as well as experimental and quasi-experimental designs. The 'new public health' model, which has been embraced all over the world since the 1980s, however, has meant that public health has had to widen its reach to embrace methods from the social sciences.

The central place occupied by ideas such as 'community action', 'supportive environments', or 'lifestyle' in recent public health discourse and debate has encouraged all public health researchers to look to the social science disciplines for new ways to explore those issues. In the last few years, that broadening of the public health researcher's methodological repertoire has even included innovations from the humanities.

In the context of the current academic climate, this book aims to provide students and practitioners of public health with a quick and accessible overview of the major methods contributing to the study of public health today. We attempt to summarise the way in which actual social behaviour and cultural influences on health have been (but also *might be*) studied. Towards the end of the book we introduce some of the major innovations that might aid public health research in the future: the methodological innovations from recent social science developments and from the humanities. Our focus has been on methods designed principally to study people — to examine lives or lifestyles rather than programs or services.

The book begins with an introduction to the history of public health *vis-à-vis* the methods that arose during that history. We have tried to show how each of the methods discussed in the rest of our book arose because of special questions pursued by particular professional cultures that were faced by specific population health problems. Knowing where our research methods come from helps us to make a more informed choice about where to use them now.

We then discuss the methods favoured by quantitative interests in public health research: surveys, epidemiological work, randomised control trials, and other outcome measures. The middle sections of the book devote themselves to methods more frequently preferred in clinical, behavioural, and social sciences circles: interviews and focus groups, but also secondary and meta-analysis. The book concludes with two chapters that examine innovations that have come exclusively from the social sciences and humanities: ethnography, action research, and semiotic and other text-based analyses.

Each of the specifically methodological chapters begins with a general introduction to the use and definitions of each method. We then discuss a variety of studies that have employed these methods in a central way. Following that discussion, we identify and assess the advantages and disadvantages of each method. We then outline some practical principles to be borne in mind when attempting to use the method under discussion. Finally we discuss some of the important ethical issues that the public health researcher needs to consider when employing the method.

The methods chapters all contain boxed summaries of important points, which can be used for quick chapter review by individual readers or as overheads for further group discussion, critique, and analysis. A list of recommended reading concludes each chapter, on the understanding that each of these chapters is necessarily introductory in its scope and aim.

We have assumed that the book will be a starting point for review of the methods that have become the cornerstone of public health research. But we have also assumed that readers will not simply want to confine themselves to the 'tried and true'. Rather we believe that they will also want to be introduced to methodological approaches that will equip them for a new millennium of developments in this exciting interdisciplinary field. To that end, this book reviews not only contemporary methods and debates, but also those emerging as future possibilities.

We have been ably and cheerfully assisted by our friend, colleague, and research assistant Sophie Hill, who for nearly a year worked tirelessly, searching for and retrieving the most representative, but also the most esoteric, literature in our broad subject area. Bronwyn Bardsley and Beth Robertson assisted in the typing and final preparation of the manuscript, a task they have happily performed for us on several other occasions. We extend our thanks to these friends for their work.

We also acknowledge the assistance of a small Australian Research Council grant, as well as a grant from the School of Sociology and Anthropology at La Trobe University. This financial assistance was crucial to our employment of Sophie and also in providing support for innumerable costs incurred in what turned out to be a major search of the public health research literature of the last ten years.

Jeanne Daly, Allan Kellehear, and Michael Gliksman
Melbourne
November 1996

CHAPTER 1

History, Public Health, and Research Methods

Imagine the sudden outbreak of a new disease. As public health researchers, we have available to us a range of methods for studying such a disease. After running tests for a disease organism, we might conduct epidemiological surveys to monitor the outbreak. We may use a randomised control trial to study the effect of treatment or prevention efforts. Especially if the disease is difficult to treat, we may use surveys or personal interviews to learn about the way it impacts on people's lives. The community groups that are most affected may significantly influence the cultural meaning attached to the disease. Here in-depth interviews are useful. Indeed, in coming to grips with the disease, we may need to conduct a series of studies using a variety of research methods, all of which fall squarely in the field of public health.

But public health researchers study more than just outbreaks of disease. Present-day public health includes issues as diverse as the prevention of disease and the empowerment of community groups. This diversity calls for an equally large, and sometimes confusing, array of research methods. It is now well understood that researchers need to choose the most appropriate method of analysis for the particular public health problem being studied. To make this choice, public health researchers need an overall methodological understanding, including the capacities and limitations of the range of available methods.

A problem that often confronts experienced health researchers as well as beginners is that research methods tend to be locked into academic disciplines, isolated from each other. Public health researchers will often have been trained in just one discipline and one set of research approaches. Indeed, only a brave researcher will claim to be confident using a research method that is the tool-of-trade of another academic discipline. And if we do stray over into the methodological preserve of other disciplines, the question remains whether we can do justice to its methods.

One way out of this impasse is to see public health as a multidisciplinary field, with researchers from different academic disciplines contributing their specialised skills to a research team. The problem experienced by many researchers working in multidisciplinary teams is that we find ourselves in a 'Tower of Babel'. Researchers from different disciplines speak different languages, based on quite different interpretations of what counts as rigorous research.

The ideal solution would be for the public health researcher to move beyond disciplinary boundaries, gaining methodological skills in a range of disciplines. This is a daunting task. In the meantime, there is no substitute for learning to speak a range of research languages with at least enough fluency to be able to join colleagues from other disciplines in choosing a research path.

Clearly a single text cannot teach the fine detail of all public health research methods. That is not the aim of this text. The first task that we have set ourselves is to describe selected public health research methods in terms of what they offer researchers, and to evaluate their contribution. Our aims are to map out the areas in which a particular research method makes an undisputed contribution and to draw attention to those areas where it may have strayed beyond methodologically defensible boundaries.

The need for a historical understanding

Public health does not exist in a vacuum, and our research methods did not just appear out of the blue. In public health today, we stand on the shoulders of those who went before us developing research methods to deal with past health crises. Each of these methods carries specific assumptions about health, the cause of disease, and the relationship between disease and society. Methods were found useful in the past not just because they contributed to knowledge but also because of the social value attached to that kind of knowledge at the time. This is something we tend to forget, and indeed, it is not a comfortable notion. Life would be much easier if research methods were value-free, delivering objective, rational knowledge about disease, irrespective of social context.

The second purpose of the book is, therefore, to develop a critical understanding of the assumptions that inform our choice of a research method. A good way of understanding both the assumptions made and the social function served by a research method is to see the method in historical context. From this we can develop a *methodological* understanding of a research method's contribution. If we also take account of the way in which the method has developed over time in response to changing circumstances, we may even, by extrapolation, be able to predict where it will go in the future.

We now turn to a historical account of public health research methods. The early history was dominated by the search for a scientific approach to public health. In the eighteenth century, the political context of social reform was intimately related to 'shoe leather' epidemiology and the use of the social survey. In the bacteriological era (during the nineteenth and early twentieth centuries), infectious disease epidemiology took over. After the Second World War, prevention of chronic disease dominated the agenda, and epidemiological methods developed and diversified. In the 1970s, the evaluation of health care became an important issue in the face of rising health-care costs. In recent times, methods focusing on the social context of health and illness have returned to prominence. In the following sections of this chapter, we deal with each of these stages in turn.

Early history and the search for science

Traditionally public health has been concerned with epidemics, not surprisingly, given the devastating effect of diseases like the plague. The problem was the difficulty of predicting epidemics and of preventing their occurrence or spread. One of the earliest contributors to the study of epidemics was Hippocrates, who urged physicians to study the environmental factors contributing to epidemics, including the air, the water, and the place in which a city was located (Hippocrates, quoted in Buck et al. 1988: 18–19). The disease itself was seen as the result of divine intervention — and this is notoriously difficult to study! A research focus on disease causation only came into prominence with the rise of modern science.

The interest in science grew out of the achievement of physicists such as Isaac Newton. Using measurement and mathematical calculation, Newton defined laws of cause and effect, which allowed scientists to predict the behaviour of objects as diverse as cannon balls, pumps, and the planets. The attraction of this science was twofold. First, the laws were universal, applying to all mechanical systems. Second, the science was very useful, leading to the invention of all sorts of machines and technologies.

Some researchers, inspired by physics, tried to apply these ideas to the study of health and illness. These efforts took two distinct forms, both of which remain with us to this day. The first, closely following Newtonian physics, reduced the problem to its constituent parts in the search for laws of cause and effect. Thus the body became a machine: the heart was seen as a pump, the stomach as a churn, and the bones and tendons as levers. This reductionist approach extended knowledge — take, for example, Harvey's study of the circulation of blood. But the body turned out to be an extremely complex machine, and there was little increase in control over disease. Thus there was room for a second approach — one that turned its attention to natural and social environments, measuring aspects of people's lives as they related to disease.

For centuries, cities and towns had kept records of people and property. Originally, bills of mortality may well have served the purpose of warning the wealthy to leave town as an epidemic emerged. Statistics, literally, were a measure of the social and economic resources of a state; 'vital statistics' reflected the health of its population (Shyrock 1961: 95). Surveillance data on health were a valuable resource, providing a range of observations that far exceeded what individual researchers could hope to collect.

In 1662 in England, John Graunt used mortality surveys to conduct an early cross-sectional study, comparing death rates in different populations. From mathematical deductions, he showed, for example, that urban populations had a higher death rate than rural populations. Then, as now, the problem was to know what to do about it. Graunt commented that the accuracy of his deductions depended upon the accuracy of the data collected. This issue, at least, could be addressed. In 1713 Jakob Bernouille developed a theory of a calculus of probability. This and subsequent studies of the life expectancy of various population groups proved useful to companies involved in providing life insurance and voluntary health insurance (Shyrock 1961: 95).

An early example of the use of surveillance data to assess the effectiveness of an intervention occurred in 1721 in Boston, during an outbreak of smallpox. Vaccination as a means of preventing the disease was known about, but was still contentious. The Reverend Cotton Mather and Zabdiel Boylston monitored the introduction of smallpox vaccination, analysing mortality statistics using a simple calculus of probabilities. They demonstrated that people who had been inoculated were less susceptible to the disease than those who had not been (Shyrock 1961: 95). Here, at last, was a way of controlling the spread of infection. But despite the development of vaccines, disease organisms had not yet been identified. Mather was a puritan priest who was also an authority on witchcraft. He would not have viewed the material aspects of life as being separate from the spiritual aspects. However, the State did not collect statistics on the moral aspects of people's lives because this was the territory of the Church.

The era of social reform

Public health, as an institution, might never have gone beyond these isolated efforts were it not for the French Revolution, during which the king was replaced as the source of legitimate power by the people or 'society'. Government 'for the common good' included the State's role as protector of the people's health. The State in France drew on science to analyse national resources, and scientists rose to positions of power in the State administration. The collection of statistics took on a new vigour, leading to studies of epidemics, the effectiveness of remedies, and the quality of mineral waters. At the same time, Marie Jean Antoine Nicolas Caritat de Condorcet advocated State support for social science, which was committed to applying scientific methods to the study of societal questions (Heilbron 1995: 109, 131).

The concept of health that arose during the French Revolution was overtly political (see Foucault 1973). The assumption was that people living under conditions of liberty, equality, and fraternity would be free of disease. Since the State was responsible for both political freedom and good health, it was proposed that doctors should be employed by the State and be encouraged to turn their attention away from disease to the study of health, including minute observation of society. In effect, instead of doctors and priests, there would be a 'therapeutic clergy', including lay people, who would preach what we might now call a health promotion message:

> after a detailed study of the whole country, a set of health regulations would have to be drawn up that would be read 'at service or mass, every Sunday and holy day', and which would explain how one should feed and dress oneself, how to avoid illness, and how to prevent or cure prevailing disease (Foucault 1973: 25–6).

With the counter-revolution of 1793, doctors (and priests) had their privileges partially restored. The emphasis on observation and measurement remained, but it was confined to hospitals rather than the community, and applied to individuals rather than populations. Dating from this period, medicine and public health had divergent agendas: medicine developed methods primarily appropriate for the study of disease in hospital populations; public health studied health in the community. Thus the first schism — the schism between medicine and public health — was set in place (White 1991).

However, the study of public health was becoming more scientific. In 1800, argues Johan Heilbron (1995: 132), French science led the world, and statistical methods provided a sound foundation for this growth. Pierre Simon Laplace published his calculus of probabilities in 1810, and in 1840 Jules Gavarret published the first book on medical statistics, which included tables for the calculation of confidence limits to address the problem of sources of error in measurement. Laplace called attention to the potential of statistical methods in analysing medical work. Pierre-Charles-Alexandre Louis took up this task, advocating what he called the 'numerical method', based on exact observation, classification, and measurement of clinical data.

In order to evaluate the effectiveness of treatment, Louis proposed setting up an adapted experiment based on two populations, selected 'indiscriminately', with only one being subjected to an intervention. One intervention studied was blood-letting. By comparing the outcomes of the two groups, the study demonstrated that blood-letting was ineffective (Louis 1835). Louis could be excused for thinking that this was useful information about a very common procedure: in 1824 alone, 33 million leeches were imported into France (Wulff 1976: 120).

The revolutionary ideas of social reform spread like wildfire through Europe and North America, and knowledge of the new numerical methods spread with them. But for over a century, medicine turned a deaf ear. Perhaps Louis's achievement in demonstrating the ineffectiveness of blood-letting was unwelcome at a time when there was little in the way of alternative medical treatments. The message was, however, heard by those who were trying to study disease in the community in a systematic way: the epidemiologists. Those who slogged on foot through areas plagued by epidemic illness earned the title of 'shoe leather' epidemiologists. Among them was John Snow. In 1855 he published a treatise on cholera, mapping the location of cases of cholera in an outbreak in London. He demonstrated that the outbreaks centred around a well in Broad Street. By removing the handle of the pump, he effected a remarkably simple preventive measure. Field epidemiology entered public health history.

The early epidemiologists could not experiment by exposing people to infectious disease. Instead, they relied on meticulous study of naturally occurring disease outbreaks. Snow was, however, alert to the possibility of natural experiments — 'happily adapted' situations in which two sites could be compared, only one of which was exposed to a potential cause of disease. He noted that there were two independent water-supply systems to a section of London, drawing their water from the Thames at different sites, only one of which was polluted with sewerage. By classifying the cholera deaths according to the source of the water supply, he demonstrated that the rate of cholera deaths from the polluted water supply was nine times higher. Despite this impressive difference, Snow felt that careful proof was needed:

> I had no reason to doubt the correctness of the conclusions I had drawn from the great number of facts already in my possession, but I felt that the circumstances of the cholera-poisoning passing down the sewers into a great river, and being distributed through miles of pipes, and yet producing its specific effects was a fact of so startling a nature, and of so vast importance to the community, that it could not be too rigidly examined or established on too firm a basis (Snow 1855).

Like Louis, Snow found that his studies had little effect. Rigorous scientific proof is still seen as the axle on which the wheel of public health reform turns. But it is one thing to produce facts of startling clarity; it is another to have them acted upon. Science, it seems, is important, but not important enough. The way in which a problem is perceived depends upon the social and political climate of the time. At the time of Snow's studies, public health disclosures of this kind were fraught with political implications in a social system under the pressure of change.

In 1848 Rudolf Virchow investigated a typhus epidemic in Upper Silesia, a province in Prussia, where a famine was raging (Trostle 1986: 45). On the basis of analysis of health statistics and his own observation, he argued that the only effective way of preventing disease was to bring about social and political change that would ensure freedom and prosperity. Virchow drew his inspiration from the studies of Friedrich Engels, friend and patron of Karl Marx. Engels had been sent to England to work in his father's factories in Manchester. Instead, he observed how people were living, documenting environmental toxins from factories, infectious disease related to poor housing, lack of nutrition, industrial accidents, and a variety of occupational diseases. While substantiating his argument with analysis based on mortality statistics, Engels also provided detailed description of the 'cattle sheds for human beings' in which people were living:

> In one of these courts there stands directly at the entrance, at the end of a covered passage, a privy without a door, so dirty that the inhabitants can pass into and out of the court only by passing through foul pools of stagnant urine and excrement . . . If any one wishes to see in how little space a human being can move, how little air — and such air! — he can breathe, how little of civilisation he may share and yet live, it is only necessary to travel hither (Engels 1958 (1844): 582–4).

Both Virchow and Engels wrote moving narrative accounts of their observations, supported by epidemiological evidence. Their work may be seen as foreshadowing the use of multiple methods, including powerful narrative accounts. They had a revolutionary aim. Engels warned: '"War to the mansion, peace to the cottage" — is a watchword of terror which may yet ring through the land. Let the wealthy beware.' (Engels, 1844: 332).

Contributing to the sense of social unrest that marked the mid-nineteenth century were the surveys that had taken the professional and amateur research world by storm (McGregor 1957). Survey skills were fostered by various professional organisations committed to statistical studies, including the London Epidemiological Society and the National Association for the Promotion of Social Science. Nancy Krieger points to the close relationship between the two disciplines (1994: 892). Sociology developed out of empirical research on social inequality, with epidemiology providing an important testing ground for social theories about the influence of society on health.

The State itself set up agencies for conducting the census as well as surveys of anything from natural resources and the weather to the diet of labouring people. Local statistical and philosophical societies conducted surveys into conditions in their towns. There were statistical comparisons of disease in towns with and without proper sewerage; other studies exposed the relationship between disease, housing, and occupation (McGregor 1957: 152). In 1842 Edwin Chadwick, a civil servant, published a comprehensive report titled *General Report on the Sanitary Conditions of the Labouring Classes of Great Britain*.

These social surveys produced systematic information on the social costs of industrial life. Under pressure, the State responded with a series of reform measures, which were only partially enforced. As the century drew to a close, there was a clear perception that the wealthy would have to pay a substantial social ransom to protect the country from the threat of socialism (McGregor 1957). In this political atmosphere, the great public health reforms of the nineteenth century were acted upon, bringing sewerage to the slums and a living wage to working people.

With the advent of these reforms, surveys linking social class and disease were eclipsed. This development was reinforced by the discovery of specific disease agents. Thus the second schism developed: epidemiology parted company with the social sciences, which continued to focus on the social context of disease.

The bacteriological era

Progressively over the nineteenth century, bacteriology and virology identified the organisms responsible for infectious diseases. The history of malaria demonstrates the variety of effective public health responses that followed. Treatment of malarial fevers by quinine was well established in the nineteenth century. Then, in 1897, Ronald Ross identified the malarial parasite in the stomach of the anopheles mosquito. Mosquito nets around beds became a common sight, swamps were drained, and anti-larval measures were instituted. After the Second World War, DDT insecticides and new preventative medication (primaquine) further diversified prevention and treatment options. The combined effect of these measures was evident in the increased industrial development of tropical countries.

The science of the laboratory was central to identifying the microscopic agents causing disease. Here, at last, was a way of breaking the problem down into constituent parts and asserting control over each in turn. The organisms were isolated and studied under laboratory conditions. Epidemiology was used to plan and evaluate interventions in the field. The public health interventions that followed were effective, cheap, and easy. Control over disease was now possible without the complex social and administrative reforms of earlier times. The marriage of the laboratory and epidemiology brought some spectacular results, none more so than the vaccine that put paid to the poliomyelitis epidemic of the 1950s. Developed and tested on laboratory animals, the Salk vaccine was then tested on human populations. The trial of the vaccine used an experimental trial design (Francis et al. 1955). Nearly 750 000 primary-school children were administered the vaccine or a placebo on a random basis, with investigators being blinded to which children belonged in each group. Laboratory tests confirmed disease incidence. They showed that the vaccine was 80–90 per cent effective in preventing poliomyelitis. The vaccine was immediately distributed, but an emergency ensued when there was an outbreak of poliomyelitis in a small number (sixty-one) of those vaccinated. The outbreak was traced to one manufacturer, and it was predicted that less than 100 cases would result from the vaccine already distributed (Langmuir 1963). Vaccination went ahead.

It has been argued that the direct savings from the Salk and then the Sabin vaccine are greater than the entire global (and considerable) expenditure on medical research (Larkins 1996). Not surprisingly, the methods that contributed to this success became enshrined in the public health consciousness. The experimental design of the double-blind randomised control trial earned the reputation of the scientific 'gold standard' for the evaluation of interventions (see chapter 5).

It is worth noting here that the language of the laboratory pervades the accounts of the community trial. The 'subjects' were viewed as little different from laboratory specimens, although parents did have to consent to participation. However, by the time of the HIV/AIDS epidemic, such trials had become contentious, requiring more careful negotiation of ethical issues both with trial participants and with the community.

Chronic disease and complexity

Concern about chronic disease came to the fore during the Second World War. Chronic disease is marked by slow progression and long duration, but according to Barrett-Connor (1979) this also applies to some infectious diseases such as tuberculosis. With infectious disease, however, there is more likely to be a microbial agent, a specific treatment, and quick responses. With chronic disease, the cause is likely to be unknown and to be associated with a variety of factors. This poses special methodological problems.

Chronic disease required researchers to return to the community to examine the social origins of disease, but this time the focus was to be on specific social agents of disease: smoking, diet, and exposure to harmful substances, including occupational exposures (Buck et al. 1988: 90). Observational methods were refined and developed to address this new challenge (see chapters 3 and 4).

A classic study of chronic disease causation is that of Richard Doll and A. Bradford Hill, based on 2370 cases of lung cancer collected in 1948–49. In a case-control design, lung cancer cases were compared with a largely comparable groups of non-cancer patients, demonstrating a 'real association' between lung cancer and smoking (Doll & Hill 1950). In 1964, they reported a ten-year observational study on a cohort of 59 600 British doctors. Smoking was found to have a 'pronounced' association with lung cancer and a range of other diseases. They concluded: 'One of the most striking characteristics of British mortality in the last half-century has been the lack of improvement in the death rate of men in middle life. In cigarette smoking may lie one prominent cause' (Doll & Hill 1964: 1467). Many researchers refused to accept the results. Perhaps this is attributable to the suspicion with which many researchers regard non-experimental epidemiological methods, or to the influence of the tobacco industry, or both.

Studies of heart disease confront a 'web of causation', which brings with it the need to take account (mathematically) of a range of social and other health-related phenomena in the community. Jeremy Morris stressed the importance of multiple causation in his classic 1957 text, *Uses of Epidemiology*. He and his co-researchers examined 687 drivers and male conductors working on London Transport buses in the late 1950s (Morris et al. 1966). Five years later they re-examined them.

Forty-seven had developed ischaemic heart disease. They found that the probability of heart disease was increased by a family history of the disease, cigarette smoking, obesity, and short stature. The study is, however, better known for its alluringly simple demonstration that bus conductors (who exercise as part of their work) have lower rates of heart disease than bus drivers.

The problem for studies of chronic disease is that the disease may only become evident many years after the behaviour that 'caused' it. Once the disease is present, it is uncommon for researchers to have access to adequate and reliable data from the past on those aspects of people's lives that might be implicated. Prospective studies deal with this problem by identifying a population, or cohort, for study and monitoring it for the occurrence of disease over time. The study population has to be stable and large enough to allow adequate statistical analysis of subgroups for each possible risk factor.

The classic cohort design is that of the Framingham study. In 1949 researchers started collecting extensive health data from a random sample of 6507 people, two-thirds of the population of Framingham, Massachusetts. It showed that high blood pressure, high plasma cholesterol and cigarette smoking are predictors of coronary risk but the investigators acknowledged that they could only demonstrate 'guilt by association' (Dawber at al. 1963).

The methodological difficulties of both collecting and analysing data from such a vast study are numerous, as are the costs. The information gained is not simple to interpret. Populations with increased 'risk factors' are identified as having a higher probability of developing the disease. Preventative interventions must change the behaviour of the 'at risk' group, reducing the probability of the disease occurring in the future. But would these preventative interventions be effective, first, in changing people's behaviour and, second, in reducing mortality? It seems reasonable simply to assume these benefits.

Questionnaire-based survey methods (see chapter 2) provided one convenient way of collecting individual data on health behaviour and other aspects of social life. Census methods were used to gather data on disease rates in different populations. However, when these were applied to a problem as complex as mental health, methodological problems emerged. Kramer (1957) wrote a telling critique of studies that demonstrated the relationship between social class and mental health, drawing on data from a psychiatric census of people under treatment on a particular day. The problem, argued Kramer, was that the rate at which disease develops in a group (incidence) is not the same as the rate that is measured in a census (prevalence). The people with a particular mental disorder under treatment on a given day represent not only the incidence of that disorder but also the availability of treatment facilities. Moreover, the people receiving treatment in various facilities, and the time they stay there, is further determined by a series of medical, social, economic, environmental, personal, familial, educational, legal, and administrative factors. Any intervention should be based on an understanding of both prevalence and incidence, and better agreement on what counts as a case. The mediating effect of social and political factors must be addressed, and this would require the participation of psychiatrists, psychologists, and social scientists in the study.

Under the impetus of such studies, the old infectious disease epidemiology gave way to a new epidemiology focused on diseases of ageing, mental health, and injuries (Gordon 1950). Epidemiological methods diversified and improved. The focus on risk factors produced a range of methodologically sophisticated studies, which occupied safe political ground. The underlying assumption, however, was that people in 'at risk' populations would respond to the information on prevention by changing their behaviour. As later sections will show, this was a rather optimistic assumption.

The modern era and evaluation of medical care

In the 1970s governments worldwide became concerned that the costs of health care were escalating without a matching gain in population health. The chief culprit was medical care. The challenge was to evaluate medical interventions, assessing both costs and effectiveness, so that only effective interventions would be funded. Louis would have rejoiced as Archie Cochrane in the United Kingdom promoted the randomised control trial as 'a very beautiful technique' for evaluating medical practice (Cochrane 1971: 22). By bringing together the concerns of medical care and the epidemiological methods of public health, some *rapprochement* between the two disciplines was brought about — a partial healing of the century-old schism (White 1991).

Two problems had to be overcome. The first was a proliferation of trials with inadequate statistical power to reach firm conclusions. The other was that trials compare interventions in terms of health outcomes, and some of these were difficult to measure.

Tom Chalmers in the USA addressed the first problem. He argued that many trials appeared to give negative results only because they lacked statistical power. By tracing published and unpublished studies within a given field and combining their data, a meta-analysis could be conducted with more reliable results (see chapter 10). Not surprisingly, trials of clinical practice were highly effective in evaluating childbirth interventions: mortality rates in mother and child could be measured. Childbirth is also a time-limited process, often occurring in an institution in which the quality of the 'product' (the infant) can be measured. The most extensive collection of trials and meta-analyses of the results is also in the field of interventions in pregnancy and childbirth (Enkin et al. 1995). This has recently led to the establishment of the International Cochrane Collaboration, named after Archie Cochrane, which maintains a database of systematic reviews of research on the effects of health care in all areas of practice.

The need for a more refined outcome measure was the second problem. Canadian George Torrance argued that what mattered was to measure not only the years of life saved or the change in a patient's health state, but also the value that society attaches to these outcomes (Torrance 1976). This could be determined by asking people to weigh up the various health outcomes resulting from a procedure and by adjusting the number of life years gained in terms of the quality of that life (see chapter 6). When this procedure was used in the case of neonatal intensive care for low-birth-weight infants, the results had highly contentious implications for health policy. Infants with very low birth weights (below 1000 grams) had lower states of health, so that the net economic cost per quality-adjusted life year gained was 17.5 times that of infants with slightly higher birth weights (1000–1500 grams) (Boyle et al. 1983). Studies such as these raise social and ethical questions about resource-allocation, for which epidemiology alone does not have the answers.

The schism with the social sciences

Epidemiologists commonly describe their method as the 'basic science' of public health. The claim to being a basic science was hard won, relying on the argument that epidemiological studies have the same degree of control over disease that the basic science studies attain in the laboratory. This claim could, however, also serve as a strategy for excluding other disciplines, such as the social sciences, from the public health field. The problem is worth addressing because it may stand in the way of recognising the contribution to public health of research methods developed primarily in the social sciences.

We take the social sciences to be those disciplines that focus their study on the relationship between individuals and the institutions and society in which they live. They include sociology, social psychology, anthropology, and others. These disciplines appear not to have been unduly perturbed by the claims of epidemiology. They have produced a substantial literature on health and society, sometimes published in public health journals, but more often in the journals of their disciplines and in multidisciplinary journals such as *Social Science and Medicine*. Being of a more theoretical bent, their contribution includes critical analysis of the whole notion of 'basic' science.

What then is a basic science? How does 'hard' science, associated with the 'natural sciences', differ from 'soft' social science methods? Not at all, argues Hedges (1987). He points out that there are direct parallels between the methods of the social sciences and the methods of physics. The cumulative effect of empirical studies in the social sciences compares very favourably with that of physics (let alone epidemiology). In demonstrating his point, Hedges made use of statistical methods for synthesising quantitative research. Indeed, many of the standard statistical procedures valued by epidemiologists were developed in sociology, in interaction with statistics (Clogg 1992).

Admittedly, Hedges was referring to quantitative studies. It is qualitative sociology that most often troubles the 'basic' scientist. Qualitative methods are based on the analysis of text and are reported in a careful argument, using words rather than numbers. Data often come from in-depth personal interviews or from discussion in focus groups (see chapters 7 and 8). Analysis takes the form of careful argument, and this narrative account may appear startlingly different from the comparatively terse accounts of trial or survey studies. Despite the difference in format, methodological rigour is given full weight, and there is no reason to believe that the knowledge gained from such studies does not make an important contribution to the science of public health.

Perhaps even more 'troublesome' are postmodern approaches. In the postmodern world, it is argued, 'grand narratives' of truth are obsolete; the focus is on 'discourses', texts, or readings, among a diversity of other discourses in a field of contending values. This approach serves two purposes. First, it frees us from the constraints of 'gold standard' methods, allowing us to be innovative in the research we conduct and to draw on the broad field of approaches used in cultural studies and social studies (see chapter 12). Second, the postmodern approach allows the notion of 'hard' science to be critically analysed.

For the past 200 years we have believed that a science based on systematisation and unifying laws was the path to universal truth and progress in the modern world. But all knowledge, including medical and epidemiological knowledge, is socially constructed in the sense that the social institutions we live in will have an inevitable effect on what we regard as a fact. Data themselves, as Krieger argues, are a social product fraught with political considerations:

> No data bases have ever magically arrived, ready made, complete with pre-defined categories and chock full of numbers. Instead, their form and content reflect decisions made by individuals and institutions, and, in the case of public health data, embodying underlying beliefs and values about what it is we need to know in order to understand population patterns of health and disease. In other words, data are a social product, and are neither a gift passively received from an invisible donor nor a neutral collection of allegedly inevitable facts . . . they cost money . . . For the funds to be released, whether from the public or private sector, people in control of these resources must consider the data to be worthwhile and capable of addressing questions that they need answered. Conversely, if they do not believe the information is necessary (or fear it may run contrary to their interests), odds are that monies to support and maintain the collection of these data will not be forthcoming. Because justification of these decisions often is framed by prevailing theories of disease causation, it is important to analyse how these theories can influence the content of public health data bases and thereby affect both public health research and its conclusions (Krieger 1992: 413–14).

Public health history shows that the research problems we perceive, the methods we choose, and the interventions that succeed are also mediated by the social and political context of the time. What, then, should we call 'basic' science? This problem should not, however, be taken to mean that researchers are freed from the responsibility of doing rigorous research. What it indicates is the need for reflective and critical understanding of what we do and how we do it.

Social science research provides its own contribution to public health, but in addition, a *rapprochement* between epidemiology and the social sciences could lead to research strategies in which each discipline brings its special skills to bear on the same health problem. We will, therefore, outline a few areas of epidemiological research in which the social sciences make an important contribution to devising better public health interventions.

One example is the study by Oakley (1985). Her meta-analysis of six observational studies and nine randomised control trials (supplemented by the evidence of another twenty-three related trials) demonstrated that the relatively simple intervention of social support during pregnancy could reduce the incidence of low birth weight in infants, overcoming the effect of low social class on both mortality and morbidity. This has direct implications for the cost of caring for infants handicapped as a result of perinatal problems. Oakley argued that by ignoring a social perspective, previous researchers had failed to recognise this strong evidence in the literature.

Social science skills also come to the fore in areas in which public health interventions have failed to reach their goal. Smoking cessation provides a good example. Despite fine epidemiological evidence and carefully targeted campaigns, which brought some decline in smoking rates, one in six deaths in the USA is still attributable to smoking (Anon. 1992). Attempts to find the answer to the problem by using methods based on exact measurements of defined variables were described by Chapman (1993) as 'unravelling gossamer with boxing gloves'. What was required were additional studies using more interpretive approaches, oral history, and discourse-analysis to make the 'complex processes such as the natural course of smoking cessation more transparent' (Chapman 1993: 432).

The problem with 'non-compliance' with preventative programs, including cancer-screening, is that the benefits of these interventions are lost not only to the individual but also to the community. But why should people not see the rationality of changing their behaviour? Here researchers have found it useful to take account of what are called 'lay' views of health, which may differ in important aspects from the medical or epidemiological view. In women's health, for example, there are clear 'strains and tensions' between a narrow biomedical model and women's more inclusive perceptions of health in all its diversity, with women even claiming the right to participate in the setting of their own health agendas (Ruzek 1993). This notion of working with a community is nothing new to the social scientist.

Vulnerable community groups with persistent health problems represent a particularly difficult field of study. Intervention programs based on informing members of the results of research are notoriously ineffective. It is not lack of knowledge but something more subtle that accounts for the problem. This is where the flexibility of qualitative methods enables researchers to be innovative in getting to know a community, learning about its values, and negotiating acceptable ways of bringing about change (see chapter 11). An example that illustrates this well is the description written by Franks (1989) of how she worked with an Australian Aboriginal community on the prevention of petrol-sniffing.

These studies do not replace epidemiological methods but complement them. In the political context of the 1990s, a *rapprochement* between the social sciences and epidemiology seems inevitable. In the past, the social science emphasis on social inequality was politically destabilising. Now, with increased concern about costs and effectiveness, a more detailed understanding of community views is an essential ingredient in an effective public health program. Communities have also become more politically active and commonly demand to be consulted in the planning and conduct of the research in which they participate. In this context, an overall research strategy that is capable of addressing a health problem from a variety of complementary perspectives is well advised.

Where to now for public health method?

The lesson to be learnt from the history of public health is that there are as many methods as there are problems. While any one time period may strongly favour a particular set of issues and associated methods, there is much to be said for having access to the full range of approaches. The public health researcher needs to engage in a more sophisticated methodological debate about what is to count as scientific rigour, and even about what is to count as the proper object of public health research.

Diversity of methods is not an indication of methodological immaturity. For some researchers, 'science' will still include only those techniques that occur in the laboratory, involving the collection of 'objective' data to test specific hypotheses under highly controlled conditions. But as we move from the management of disease by pharmaceutical solutions towards prevention of disease in the community, our research field must move out of the laboratory. In the process, we lose control over the research environment (the disease to be studied is in people and not in a test tube) and we have to take account of many interactive contributing factors in the way in which people live their lives. This is where we have to turn to a range of other methods. Chronic diseases such as cancer, asthma, arthritis or any number of new and existing chronic conditions may claim our attention and call for a range of epidemiological approaches. In order to understand the manifestations of disease in the community, we need to pay more attention to the social context of disease. The issue here is whether, in the process of moving out of the laboratory, we are giving up 'science' for something less objective, less certain, and less likely to be effective.

The argument of this book is that we can and should be scientific about the study of all public health problems. This requires careful analysis of what we use as data, our methods of analysis, and our conclusions. We need to recognise the limitations and achievements of the full range of public health methods in order to match problem to method more effectively.

CHAPTER 2

Simple Questionnaire Surveys

Whether you know it or not, you have been a participant in a survey that is repeated at regular intervals throughout your life. No, this is not the introduction to a chapter on conspiracy theories, nor is it a failed script for 'The X Files'. At its most basic form, a survey can be defined as a study involving a group of people selected from a larger group of people. Researchers usually, and sometimes incorrectly, make the assumption that the smaller group is representative of the larger group. This smaller group (or *sample*) of the larger group (or *population*) are then observed and/or questioned on the variables of interest to the researchers. The latter is the questionnaire-based survey. If the whole population is surveyed, it is known as a census. This is the survey in which you have participated.

From the results of surveys carried out on samples drawn from a larger population, summary statistics can be used to draw inferences about the characteristics of the same variables in the population. The validity and reliability of these inferences will depend on a number of factors. The most important of these factors are how representative the sample is of the population from which it was drawn, and how accurately and comprehensively the questionnaire used gathered the information of interest.

'Validity' (also known as 'accuracy') and 'reliability' (also known as 'repeatability') are terms you will encounter frequently in public health research. Both are used to describe the quality of measurements, including those resulting from questionnaire-based surveys.

The two most important kinds of validity are 'internal' and 'external'. 'Internal validity' refers to the degree to which the sample results accurately represent the sample members' views, characteristics, or opinions of interest. If the questionnaire was well constructed and correctly administered, the results are more likely to be internally valid. 'External validity' refers to how well the sample results apply to the population from which the sample was drawn. This is also known as 'generalisability'. A survey with excellent internal validity may be misleading if the sample is not representative of the population to which you want to generalise your findings.

Reliability refers to the repeatability of results. In order to be useful, a questionnaire must be able to reproduce similar results when repeatedly used to measure the same variable in the same group. However, it is important to realise that reliability is not the same as validity or accuracy. A reliable questionnaire, like a reliable but inaccurate rifle, may miss the bull's-eye every time by a similar distance.

The accuracy or validity of a questionnaire is of utmost importance in assessing questionnaire-based surveys. The questionnaire also forms the basis of the larger class of non-experimental studies, of which questionnaire-based surveys are a part. These studies are non-experimental in the sense that the researcher does not manipulate variables of interest or factors thought to affect the outcome. The researcher 'simply' measures these factors in as valid and reliable a way as possible.

Most surveys occur at a single point in time and are therefore known as 'cross sectional' or 'prevalence' studies, although they may be repeated on several occasions as part of a follow-up or 'longitudinal' study. The simple questionnaire survey's main purpose, therefore, is to obtain a snapshot in time of a population's attitudes, health status, behaviours, or the like. If obtained correctly, such information is invaluable in providing politicians and public health officials with the good quality data that are a prerequisite for effective public health policy formulation and action.

Some examples

Many surveys attempt to assess consumer beliefs that may impact on the effectiveness of public health programs, or that give insight into health-related attitudes and behaviours. The importance of this work is difficult to overestimate. Without a clear and accurate understanding of community beliefs and priorities, resource-allocation and priority-setting within the public health arena become little more than a hit and miss affair.

In Australia Hill and others (1991) sampled 3527 men and women aged sixteen years and over in their homes to obtain insights into behavioural risk factors for cancer. A two-stage sampling technique was used. First, a house within a given census-collector's district was randomly selected. Within each household, an individual was selected according to predetermined criteria. One person was interviewed per household. The resulting sample characteristics were checked with Australian Bureau of Statistics criteria for representativeness. The questionnaire, which was developed in consultation with expert staff at the Anti-Cancer Council of Victoria, was extensively pilot-tested to ensure its validity. It was administered by trained interviewers. Four-fifths of the participants were able to nominate at least one step they could take to reduce their risk of cancer, but almost 20 per cent could not — a result of great significance to public health educators.

Lowe and others (1993) surveyed the sun-related attitudes of 3655 children in grades 7–11 from fifty-five schools in Queensland. As with Hill and others (1991), a two-stage sampling technique was used. Schools were stratified by locality and size of school. By stratification, we mean that schools were first grouped according to locality and size *before* participating schools were randomly selected from each stratum for inclusion in the survey proper. This is known as a 'stratified random sample'. The advantage of this method lies in the improved likelihood that children from different areas and different-sized schools will have an approximately equal chance of being selected for inclusion in the survey. This adds considerably to the representativeness of the sample selected.

Children in those schools were then selected for interview by predetermined criteria. Focus group discussion and comparison with other attitudinal questionnaires were undertaken to ensure that the questionnaire used was valid. The questionnaire was administered by a class teacher. (You could question the validity of this approach in comparison with using a questionnaire administrator not known to the children.) The results of the survey revealed attitudinal barriers to sun protection, especially marked among boys. These data could then be used to modify school-based sun protection programs to make them more sensitive to age and sex differences.

Patton and hordes of associated researchers (1995) used a similar two-stage sampling technique to survey the current level of drug-use and its patterns among Victorian secondary-school students. In contrast to the above study, this survey was administered by computer to ensure confidentiality, an important issue in terms of validity when controversial or emotionally charged matters are the subject of a survey. Frequent users of alcohol and tobacco were found to be the most frequent users of illegal substances, which was a finding of considerable importance to drug-use educators.

Rissel (1991) combined a survey with physical measurement to determine the association between television-viewing and obesity in adults. The research participants were 290 staff who were present at the Panther Leagues Club in Sydney over a five-day period in 1990 (just over one-third of all staff on duty at the time). There was no obvious reason why they were chosen other than that they were there and they agreed to participate. This is known as a 'convenience' sample (probably because it is convenient for the researchers). The advantages, disadvantages, and ethics of this sort of design will be discussed later; suffice to say that this study could reach no valid conclusions because of the small numbers surveyed.

The issue of validity and representativeness arises again with regard to a sample survey measuring the food consumption of parents on low incomes in the inner-city suburb of Redfern, Sydney (Buchhorn 1995). In this instance, participants were recruited from among attendees at community-activity and child-health centres. Of the sixty participants recruited, fifty-one (but only four men) completed well-validated food-frequency questionnaires. Few differences were found between the eating habits of these people and previous results gathered using the same food-frequency questionnaire among other segments of the wider community.

The use of two-stage random sampling is well established internationally. Verhaak and Tijhuis (1992) first selected a representative sample of Dutch general practitioners. All patients with whom these practitioners had contact over a three-month period who met predetermined criteria were approached. Well-established self-administered health questionnaires were used and were repeated one year later. This provided evidence on the changing prevalence of psychosocial problems among people presenting to their general practitioners both with and without overt complaints of such problems.

Surveys have been used in other areas of public health to assess the prevalence of health-associated variables. In the autumn of 1990, Link and others (1994) used random digit dialling (using randomly generated phone numbers) in the USA to survey 1507 adults in all states except Hawaii and Alaska. Respondents were asked if they had ever been homeless. Lifetime and five-year prevalence rates for homelessness were then calculated, the latter being 14 per cent. Although this seems high, it is worth considering the issue of external validity with regard to a telephone survey of homelessness. With the advent of mobile phones, will this become a less significant source of bias in future studies of the homeless?

Leigh and others (1994) collected survey questionnaire data on sexual behaviour and risk of HIV from 2058 respondents in the USA, selected by multi-stage probability methods of the type already discussed earlier in this chapter. Due to the sensitivity of the issues covered in the questionnaire, questions specifically about sexual behaviour were posed as a self-assessment questionnaire (SAQ) with anonymity assured. The authors reported a strong correlation between alcohol-use, multiple partners, and condom-use.

An SAQ was also used in Australia to assess the knowledge and practice of safe sex among homosexual men in Melbourne (Ridge, Plummer, & Minichiello 1994). However, a convenience sample of 284 men was used, recruited from gay groups, health clinics, social networks, and elsewhere. The comparatively high rate of condom-use may have resulted from the methodology used, drawing the issue of generalisability into focus. This drawback was recognised by the authors, who urged caution, especially in generalising their findings to men who have sex with other men but do not openly identify themselves as homosexual and socialise accordingly.

Boekeloo and others (1994) compared the results of surveys into HIV-risk-factor behaviours that used audio questionnaires with those that used written questionnaires. Even though both were SAQs, differences were found in the results obtained from randomly selected participants, which brings us to the issue of the advantages and disadvantages of survey methods.

Advantages and disadvantages

The overwhelming advantage of using simple questionnaire surveys as a means of gathering information, opinions, attitudes, health status, and so on lies in the method's ability to do so in a cost-efficient and timely manner. There are several potential disadvantages, but they can be minimised if care is taken in selecting the survey methods, and in the construction and administration of the survey instruments (questionnaire). It is the very features that make surveys so logistically attractive that can compromise the meaning and validity of their results.

Let us return to the telephone-based survey of prevalence of homelessness in the USA (Link et al. 1994). (After all, when you are on to a good example, why not stick to it?) Telephone surveys may not be the best approach to researching homelessness, but surely they are useful in other areas? They are quick, inexpensive, and relatively simple to administer. The use of random digit dialling seems to overcome any risk of sample selection bias. Phoning out of normal business hours, and repeated phoning if no one is home initially, seems likely to overcome any risk of bias that might occur if people were missed because they were out at work, visiting, shopping, or somewhere else at the time of the initial call. Yet this may not be so.

In Australia a comparison was made of survey results obtained by random selection from the telephone directory and the electoral rolls (Gliksman et al. 1987). The results showed that, even where the usual precautions were used, up to 31 per cent of people listed on the federal electoral rolls were inaccessible to interview by telephone. More disturbing from the viewpoint of bias and validity was the finding that those who were inaccessible to telephone contact differed from those who were accessible with regard to a number of important socio-economic and health indicators. These include employment status and self-reported health status. So it seems that the methods used will strongly affect the accuracy, validity and meaning of the results obtained. As in so many areas, cheap may also mean nasty.

Another form of survey sampling that has the advantage of simplicity and cost is the mailed or postal questionnaire. This involves (ideally) the mailing of SAQs to (ideally) a representative sample of people. The main advantages are that it enables whole populations or large samples to be surveyed in a relatively inexpensive manner. For example, a United States survey on the correlation of frequent dieting among 33 393 adolescents could not have been conducted by any other method (French et al. 1995). Not having to do face-to-face interviews or gain permission for interviews has considerable logistical advantages, not to mention cost savings. However, it should not surprise you that, as with much in life, it also confers considerable costs. An SAQ on attitudes to heart disease was mailed to a random sample of 1800 people in the Hunter Valley in New South Wales as a prelude to planning for the preventive and treatment needs of all residents in that locality (Buchhorn 1995). The overall response rate was only 56 per cent. There was further disturbing evidence that the response rate was lowest among those in the lowest socio-economic categories. Since socio-economic status is one of the strongest predictors of heart disease, this is a most serious potential source of bias. Despite this, conclusions were drawn about the needs for health promotion activity in the Hunter Valley. This is a matter we will return to when we discuss the ethics of surveys.

Some of the problems of poor response rates can be overcome by confining the use of mailed questionnaires to highly motivated groups. This was the technique used by Elliot (1995) in her survey. A food frequency questionnaire was administered by mail to a representative sample of 137 people previously diagnosed with possible or definite heart attack. She achieved a 78 per cent response rate, which suggests that, if the sample is well motivated, response rates from the use of such a logistically convenient method may be acceptable. However, again there was evidence that convenience carries a cost in bias. The self-reported information on weight and height suggested underestimation of the former. There was also a suggestion that those whose diet might have been 'better' from the perspective of heart disease were more likely to respond than others.

Another postal survey, into postnatal depression, showed that this method suffered from an underrepresentation of young mothers, single mothers, and women from non-English-speaking backgrounds (Astbury et al. 1994), the very people most likely to experience postnatal depression. The greatest disadvantage associated with convenience may be the underestimation of the extent and nature of the problem you are interested in. Socio-economic status and ethnic origin have both been shown to affect response rates to a postal survey on faecal occult blood-screening (King et al. 1994). The authors wisely pointed out that these matters must be taken into account when planning (and, we would stress, in interpreting the results from) such surveys.

In addition to the one already discussed (Gliksman et al. 1987), several studies have directly compared the advantages and disadvantages of several survey methods. These comparisons guide us regarding the advantages and disadvantages of differing approaches to the three main areas of survey design: questionnaire construction, sampling selection, and methods of questionnaire administration.

Kooiker (1995) compared the validity of data obtained by using open-ended questions with the validity of results achieved by forcing respondents to choose among closed alternatives. Open-ended questions reduced the bias in data obtained on the prevalence of everyday illnesses, but they resulted in fewer symptoms being recorded. Quine (1985) reported that the use of a highly structured questionnaire minimised the effects of differences in the method of questionnaire administration (face-to-face, telephone, SAQ). Conversely, Boekeloo and others (1994) concluded that, where highly sensitive material is sought — such as risk behaviour in relation to HIV — an SAQ is the method most likely to yield valid results. Face-to-face questionnaires seemed more likely to meet with guarded responses. Like so much else in good-quality science, the key to choosing an appropriate survey method is just common sense.

The findings reported almost a decade earlier by Gliksman and others (1987) were reflected in the results reported by Turrell and Najman (1995). They compared the results obtained when a food-related questionnaire was administered as an SAQ (respondents having been selected from electoral rolls) with the results obtained when the questionnaire was administered face-to-face. Drawing a sample from an electoral roll and then sending the questionnaire for self-administration was shown to greatly understate the level of socio-economic inequality affecting food-related behaviour in the community about which conclusions were to be drawn.

Finally, three data-collection methods (street intercept, telephone ring-in, and focus-group discussions) — all used to gather data on drug-related matters from young illicit drug-users — were compared on the grounds of validity and cost (Spooner & Flaherty 1993). All seemed equally valid (or invalid). The main difference between them was cost, with street intercept methods, which lead to face-to-face interviews, proving to be the least expensive option.

The most important lesson to be gained from all this is that the optimum method will depend on the issues you wish to address, the sample or population you wish to study, and the resources available to you. But within those constraints, what principles can be followed to achieve the most valid results possible?

Advantages of the survey:
- It can have a relatively simple design.
- It can be inexpensive to conduct.
- Researchers are offered a choice of administration modes.

Disadvantages of survey:
- It is easy to obtain invalid results.
- It can only determine prevalence, not incidence.
- It cannot definitively answer questions of causality.

Some practical principles

It should be apparent that, in order to construct a reliable and valid survey instrument, you will need to be well acquainted with the literature of the area you wish to survey, as well as the characteristics of the population to which you wish to apply your results. Otherwise it will be very difficult either to design a valid questionnaire or to select a sample that is truly representative of the population of interest. Levy and Lermeshow (1991) have pointed out that, whether a survey is large or small, complicated or relatively simple in design, the validity or generalisability of results will largely depend on the quality of design, sample selection, and conduct of the study.

They also point out that a design must be feasible; it must be able to be completed with the resources available. This is why simple random sampling is rarely used in survey designs. In a simple random sample, each member of the population to which you wish to generalise the results has an equal chance of being chosen to form part of the sample. Think about this. If, like Guest and others (1992), you want to say something about smoking and nutrition among Australian Aborigines, is a simple random sample feasible? The population of Australian Aborigines is spread over the continent. Simple random sampling over such a geographic distribution would be very costly to implement. The researchers therefore restricted their sampling to defined geographical areas in two Victorian towns. The advantage is that the study can be done. The disadvantage is that the Aborigines in these towns cannot be regarded as completely representative of all Australia's Aboriginal population. However, systematic sampling, if done well, can yield valid results from a feasible study. For those of you who wish to delve into the technicalities of systematic sampling, Levy and Lermeshow (1991) provide a good starting point.

Some further examples will help you get a grasp of the idea. Brown and Lumley (1993) were interested in issues surrounding consumer satisfaction with antenatal services in Victoria. Surveying samples drawn from throughout Victoria would have been expensive, but surveying within restricted geographic areas might have resulted in an unrepresentative sample and invalid results. The dilemma was resolved by selecting a fixed period of time and mailing enough questionnaires to cover all births throughout Victoria during the second week of February 1989. This survey was systematic in terms of time restriction.

As pointed out earlier, the risk with systematic sampling is that it will create an unrepresentative sample. This risk was recognised by Higginbotham and others (1993) when they conducted a survey into community perceptions of heart disease risk in the Hunter Valley in New South Wales. Results of a survey that drew its sample only from the inland regions of the Valley would have been applicable only to lower socio-economic groups. The researchers therefore also deliberately sampled from higher socio-economic regions of the Valley, which increased the generalisability of their results, as well as allowing them to compare attitudinal differences between different socio-economic status groups.

In working through the issue of sample selection, one task is to ensure external validity so that the results from the sample also apply to the population from which it is drawn. The parallel task is to ensure internal validity by designing a questionnaire that collects reliable, accurate and valid results from the people in the sample. Given the number of public health settings in which questionnaire surveys are used, a detailed discussion of questionnaire construction is beyond the scope of this chapter. For those interested in pursuing this matter further, we recommend de Vaus (1990), which is included in the list of recommended readings. However, whatever questionnaire design is chosen, Sirken (1986) has pointed out the importance of developing and testing questionnaires before using them on the sample chosen.

Surveying ethics

As with all aspects of research design, 'good science' and ethical behaviour are complementary; they are not in competition. It is poor science to use methods that are likely to yield poor or unrepresentative sample response rates. It is both poor science and poor ethics to generalise results from a study that has poor validity.

This issue was clearly in the minds of Guest and others (1992) when they conducted their survey of smoking and associated health behaviours among Aboriginal Australians. To improve the participation rate, the researchers consulted with local Aboriginal community leaders, which resulted in a relatively high participation rate: 90 per cent of all Aboriginal people asked to take part.

Researchers are always on the lookout for methods to improve participation rates. Chapman and Wong (1991) presented evidence that the offer of a $1 'Scratchie' (a 'scratch-and-win' lottery card) dramatically improved survey participation rates without evidence of biasing effects. However, when evaluating the ethics of such a method, we should consider the effects that offering rewards in some studies might have on subsequent participation rates for studies that do not offer such rewards. While it may boost participation rates in those studies that can afford to offer rewards, it may reduce rates in those studies not offering rewards. If this is the case, is the offer of a reward still ethical?

The ethics of using convenience samples must also be questioned. Convenient to researchers they may be, but the results may be inaccurate and therefore invalid (Leigh et al. 1994). Buchhorn (1995) approached people through community centres to fill out food frequency questionnaires. Although the sample could not be considered representative of low-income families, results were generalised to that wider community. Is it ethical to apply such results to people whose behaviour characteristics and values may not have been represented in the sample surveyed?

Oddy and Stockwell (1995) highlighted the extent of the ethical and scientific dilemmas posed by similar problems with simple questionnaire surveys. They showed that simple questionnaire surveys, when dealing with controversial subject matter, can yield scientifically invalid results. Their study demonstrated that population surveys of alcohol-consumption account for only about 60 per cent of alcohol sold. Presumably, 40 per cent is lost through evaporation following purchase! The researchers suggested that the disparity resulted from under-reporting by respondents and undersampling of heavy and problem drinkers.

Careful questionnaire construction and administration, guarantees of confidentiality, and truly representative sampling are ethical and scientific essentials, especially when controversial or potentially embarrassing topics are being surveyed. Honig (1995) has described a practical method for ensuring confidentiality in questionnaire-based surveys, in which respondents are linked to a code number based on personal details, which remain confidential for all but the principal researchers. This technique boosts participation rates in an ethically consistent fashion.

Another ethical issue is that of informed consent. Participants have the right to be informed of the aims and methods of the study, funding sources, and the use to which the data are to be put. In this age of (hopefully) active ethics committees, it is usual for those planning surveys to consider carefully the issue of informed consent. However, there are still some areas in which the rights of survey participants may receive less than ideal levels of attention. Where studies involve children and young people, researchers sometimes positively gloat about the fact that the participants, especially children at school, 'are in an uniquely favourable setting as a captive audience' (Lowe et al. 1993). In that study (as in many others involving young people), there is no evidence that the consent of the young person was sought before attitudinal and other personal data were obtained. Would it be ethical for someone to force you to participate in a survey? If not, why would it be for others?

Recommended reading

Axelsson, G. & Helgadottir, S. 1995, 'Comparison of Oral Health Data from Self-Administered Questionnaire and Clinical Examination', *Community Dental and Oral Epidemiology*, vol. 23, pp. 365–8.

This is a good example of comparative techniques in medical surveys.

Fletcher, R.H., Fletcher, S.W., & Wagner, E.H. 1988, *Clinical Epidemiology: The Essentials*, 2nd edn, Williams & Wilkins, Baltimore.

This provides a good overview of research techniques and issues.

Grubb, A., Walsh, P., Lambe, N., et al. 1996, 'Survey of British Clinicians' Views on Management of Patients in a Persistent Vegetative State', *Lancet*, vol. 348, pp. 35–40.

This is good example of surveys in action.

Hahn, S.R., Kroenko, K., Spitzer, R.L., et al. 1996, 'The Difficult Patient: Prevalence, Psychopathology and Functional Impairment', *Journal of General Internal Medicine*, vol. 11, pp. 1–8.

This article is an example of how surveys can be conducted in difficult circumstances.

Last, J.M. 1995, *A Dictionary of Epidemiology*, 3rd edn, Oxford University Press, New York.

The title says it all.

Levy, P.S. & Lermeshow, S. 1991, *Sampling of Populations: Methods and Applications*, John Wiley & Sons, New York.

Levy and Lermeshow provide a good, if somewhat technical, overview.

McDowell, I. & Newell, C. 1987, *Measuring Health: A Guide to Rating Scales and Questionnaires*, Oxford University Press, New York.

The bible; old testament.

Sleep, J., Bullock, I., & Grayson, K. 1995, 'Establishing Priorities for Research in Education within One College of Nursing and Midwifery', *Nurse Education Today*, vol. 15, pp. 439–45.

This demonstrates how to survey arcane areas

Vaus, D. de 1990, *Surveys in Social Research*, Unwin Hyman, London.

The bible.

CHAPTER 3

Epidemiological Surveys

Epidemiology is a research discipline that interests itself in the patterns of distribution and risk factors for disease in whole populations. Epidemiological surveys are, by and large, large-scale surveys of a significant proportion of the population. Epidemiology therefore goes beyond the boundaries of traditional clinical medicine by dealing with populations rather than individuals. As a result, epidemiology is often regarded as 'the basic science' of public health practice and research.

The science of epidemiology is geared towards determining the existence of health, disease, exposures, and other possible risk factors for disease in terms of the frequency of their occurrence and the distribution of these factors throughout the population. The technique of epidemiology is to look for associations in these distributions that will give clues about which factors could be related to causes of disease or good health in that population.

The aim of such a survey is to map or chart patterns of disease, or risk factors for disease, in that population at a particular time, or to chart the changes of such patterns over a period of time. The aim may be to determine what the risk factors are and under what circumstances they operate.

Partly because such surveys are conducted among large groups, in which individual factors are 'diluted' by group experiences, the associations that are uncovered between possible exposures and outcomes are referred to as 'probabilities' or 'risks'. It is often difficult to grasp the concept that these risks are simply the probability that one group or subset with a particular attribute or exposure — compared with another sub-set either with or without certain risk factors — may or may not develop an outcome of interest. It is as though the epidemiologist, through the device of an epidemiological survey, is able to predict with greater and greater accuracy, but not with absolute certainty, the fall of a dice, the draw of a card, or the final resting point of the roulette wheel. This is a nice skill to have if you like to gamble, which is what many of us do in our lives in relation to health matters anyway.

Fletcher, Fletcher, and Wagner (1988) have pointed out that, because epidemiologists work with groups of individuals, they also work with probabilities based on those groups of individuals. Each individual may display unique genetic and environmental characteristics. Therefore one of the principle characteristics of epidemiological surveys is the way in which they adjust for the effects of many different variables and provide summary statistics. The aim is to determine whether chance could account for the associations found, or whether the associations may indicate a causative relationship. This is an important issue, and a common criticism of epidemiological surveys is that it is often too difficult to make such a determination. Are the associations found the result of chance, or do they indicate a true causative relationship?

The problem is seen most clearly when one discusses the relationship between cigarette-smoking and lung cancer or cardiovascular disease. Because many factors are involved, at both an individual and group level, proponents of cigarette-smoking suggests that it may be other factors related to cigarette-smoking that are responsible for higher rates of cancer among smokers rather than the smoking itself. Some of the arguments put forward suggest that the cause of the cancer is air pollution or certain food additives. To deal with these problems, epidemiologists have developed tests for causation to distinguish between chance and true relationships.

Epidemiology is a scientific discipline that deals with human populations rather than individuals. As such, it is not able to provide experimental proof of causation of disease in the classic sense of observing the effects of putative causative factors on outcomes, as can be done with laboratory experiments or in randomised control trials (chapter 5). Often experiments are not possible and only observational studies such as epidemiological surveys are available. Indeed, much of what we know of disease is traceable to epidemiological surveys in populations. How is it, then, that a branch of medical science that cannot provide classic proofs is able to provide useful information about disease causation?

In 1965 the British statistician A. Bradford Hill (1965) proposed a set of criteria that have become established as a test of causality. The criteria include:

1 *Temporality.* The postulated cause or risk factor should precede the outcome of interest. As you will appreciate, this is probably the most important of the tests of causality. If a potential cause or risk factor cannot be shown to precede an outcome of interest, its causal relationship must be in serious doubt. However, many epidemiological surveys are cross-sectional in nature; in other words, they are done at one particular point in time, at which both postulated causes and outcomes are measured. In these circumstances, causality can only be inferred and subsequent investigations — epidemiological or otherwise — are needed to establish the temporal relationships.

2 *Strength.* There should be a fairly strong association between the proposed risk factor and the outcome of interest.

3 *Dose response.* A larger exposure to the postulated risk factor should equate to higher rates of the outcome of interest.

4 *Reversibility.* A reduction in contact or exposure to the postulated risk factor should be associated with a declining rate of the outcome of interest.

5 *Consistency.* The association should be observed in a number of studies, in different places, circumstances, and times.

6 *Biological plausibility.* Naturally this applies to biological systems, but one might argue that psychological or sociological plausibility should carry equal weight in those fields. This is not a particularly essential test of causality. Knowledge and attitudes change over time, and what makes biological, psychological, or sociological sense at one point in time (or in one era or system of belief) may not at another.

7 *Specificity.* This is the requirement that one type of postulated exposure is associated with a particular type of outcome. Again, this is not a particularly important test of causality. It is possible for one type of exposure to be associated with several outcomes. Likewise, it may take several different sorts of exposures, possibly at different times and at different levels, to lead to a particular outcome.

8 *Analogy.* This is when similar cause-and-effect relationships to the one in question are established. For example, the fact that a disease such as kuru (a wasting brain disease in certain New Guinean tribes)

can be spread by the eating of human remains suggested the mechanism by which mad cow disease could cross species barriers. However, analogy is weak evidence for a cause- and-effect relationship.

Some examples

As mentioned previously, epidemiological surveys are primarily aimed at determining associations between putative risk factors and outcomes, thus lending themselves to a wide range of purposes within the broader discipline of public health research. This breadth of application can most clearly be seen by examining examples of the science and art of epidemiological surveys. One of the most common functions of the public health survey is that of evaluating the effectiveness of public health and intervention programs. Such programs are designed either to increase awareness of risk factors or to reduce the prevalence of such factors within the general community or a specific sub-set.

One well-known example of this evaluative function concerns the Minnesota Heart Health Programme, which is a thirteen-year research and demonstration project designed to reduce morbidity and mortality from coronary heart disease in a whole community (Luepker et al. 1988). This study matched three pairs of whole communities on the basis of size and a number of socio-demographic factors previously shown to be associated with heart disease. In other words, the researchers went to some effort to ensure they were comparing similar populations. Each pair of communities had one intervention site and one comparison site. After baseline surveys (the first in a series of surveys) of pre-existing risk, a five-to-six-year program was commenced, involving mass media, community organisations, and direct education for risk reduction. Epidemiological surveys continued during this period at all sites. Favourable changes in the incidence of most coronary heart disease risk factors were found in the study communities. By the repeated use of epidemiological surveys, longitudinal data were obtained that validated the effectiveness of community intervention strategies on a number of the criteria enunciated by Hill (1965).

Similarly, the Pawtucket Heart Health Programme used random-sample cross-sectional surveys on people aged 18–64 years. These were conducted before, during, and after education programs on coronary health (Carleton et al. 1995). This study was also able to use repeated measurement over time to adapt what was essentially a cross-sectional technique, thus providing longitudinal data on the effectiveness of community-wide intervention strategies.

The technique of repeating epidemiological surveys within a specific community was used to measure prospective changes in cardiovascular risk during a six-year multiple-risk-factor intervention study. The changes were correlated with differences in socio-demographic, psychosocial, and physiological characteristics in a sample of 221 women and 190 men, aged 25–74 years, who were included in four surveys undertaken between 1979 and 1985. This technique yielded longitudinal data that enabled the researchers to recommend specific intervention to target differences in age, socio-economic, and cultural sub-groups, with a good degree of validity (Winklcby et al. 1994).

Epidemiological surveys, used in the manner described, also enable the tracking of changes in knowledge and attitudes that might affect the relationship between certain risk factors and disease outcomes. For example, Langenhoven and others (1991) conducted a community-oriented heart disease risk factor intervention study in three distinct rural communities in South Africa, reporting on health and diet knowledge as it relates to coronary heart disease. They were able to show that dietary knowledge among their community survey group was poor. In particular, males, the young, and individuals with lower levels of education had poor levels of knowledge about the risk factors for heart disease. Following intervention — which consisted of a three-year, small media program in one community, additional interpersonal intervention among high-risk individuals in a second community, and no intervention of either nature in a 'control' community — both of the communities that received intervention demonstrated significant improvement in knowledge. The researchers were also able to correlate differences in knowledge gain with gender and education levels, providing information about those sub-groups within communities that require particular education programs.

However, all is not sweetness and light. A review of multiple interventions in middle-aged men conducted by Oliver (1992) dealt with some of the limitations of epidemiological surveys in identifying risk factors and their relationship to health. That review concluded that, after many years of study, the public health community still does not understand enough about the risk factors of coronary heart disease to know why the cardiovascular disease rate (at least in the United Kingdom, the home of the greasy fish and chip) remains resistant to community-based efforts to control it. Although not specifically stated, Oliver's article suggests that certain flaws within the methodologies of some studies may account for some unusual findings. Included among these findings is the higher rate of violence-associated deaths in an intervention group that was successful in lowering cholesterol. It was suggested by Oliver that, even though such a result defies biologically plausible explanations, it should not be dismissed or ignored just because it cannot be explained (Muldoon et al. 1990; Oliver 1991). Sometimes research provides more questions than answers.

Another major use of epidemiological surveys is to identify the health needs of a given community within a given period of time. This can include identifying or inferring needs by examining patterns of morbidity or mortality during either a single or repeated survey within a given community.

An example of this use can be found in the Busselton study, which was conducted over a number of years in Western Australia (Knuiman et al. 1994). Since 1966 the community of Busselton in Western Australia has participated in repeated cross-sectional epidemiological health surveys, all associated with health-related interventions. Every three years, health surveys of adults were conducted between the years 1966 and 1981. Measurement of health-related outcomes also occurred in late 1989. This survey was able to show that, for females, especially those aged 45–74 years, mortality rates were declining at a significantly faster rate than for males in the Busselton region. As well as providing information on the beneficial impact of intervention on survival, the study was able to identify gender-specific health needs within the community and their change over time. Such data are of considerable importance to public health planners in assessing the need for limited health resources, and in assigning or distributing these resources in the most cost-effective manner possible.

Epidemiological surveys can also be used to highlight the spectrum of disease that may result from particular exposures. For example, Viel and Richardson (1993) were able to correlate the occurrence of lymphoma, multiple myeloma, and leukaemia among male French farmers and farm labourers with pesticide exposure. After adjustment for socio-economic status, they were able to demonstrate a significant link between pesticide exposure and leukaemia mortality.

Similarly, epidemiological surveys have been used to describe the natural history of diseases. In these circumstances, the surveys are generally repeated over a period of time, following a baseline study — as with the Busselton study, the methodology of which has already been discussed. With this baseline study and repeated surveys, the researchers in the Busselton study were able to show that the mortality rates from heart disease and stroke in Australia had been falling for more than twenty years. This was believed to be due, in part, to changes in the incidence of cardiovascular disease, which in turn arose from changes in the prevalence and severity of the risk factors of cardiovascular disease. Over the course of the study, downward secular trends were observed in relation to blood pressure and smoking among men and women, while upward trends were observed in relation to body mass index in men. Mean cholesterol levels among men remained relatively constant.

If conducted over a long time, such studies can answer complex questions about the association between childhood exposures and disease in later life. The Nurse's Health Study, conducted from the Channing Laboratory at Harvard Medical School, has shown what is possible in this regard. Controlling for a number of other factors that may have influenced the outcome, one aspect of this study showed that childhood socio-economic status was related to risk of cardiovascular disease among middle-aged American women. (Gliksman et al. 1995).

Similarly, a nationally representative British sample of over 3000 men and women aged thirty-six years showed that current health problems were related to earlier life events (Kuh & Wadsworth 1993). They too were able to show that those adults who came from poorer family backgrounds, or who were least educated, experienced worse health outcomes in their adult years.

Disease trends can be predicted by similar approaches. The observation of changes over time by means of repeated epidemiological surveys allows prediction of likely disease trends in the future. An example of this approach is the Western Sydney Stroke Risk Study in the Elderly (Gliksman et al. 1994). This baseline survey among men and women aged sixty-five years and older, all of whom were residents in several retirement villages in the western metropolitan region of Sydney, established the dietary, lifestyle, medical, and socio-demographic variables that were of relevance to health outcomes. Repeated surveys each year thereafter were able to demonstrate trends in disease outcomes, allowing projections to be made into the future. Such projections are of particular interest to public health professionals who must plan resource-allocation in relation to future health-care needs.

Finally, a very powerful use of epidemiological surveys is to elucidate mechanisms of disease transmission or causation. Bailey and others (1994) were able to demonstrate a link between the processes of urbanisation and industrialisation in Massachusetts, USA, and blood lead levels among children in this state. Elevated levels of blood lead among children are of great concern, as they are associated with reduced intellectual ability and educational performance, resulting in greater risk of poverty and disease in later life. It can be seen that epidemiological surveys are a sufficiently powerful technique, if used correctly, to provide evidence in relation to environmental damage and its impact on individual and population health. In terms of wider public policy, such uses of epidemiology are likely to make a significant impact on political decision-making processes that go beyond traditional public health fields.

Advantages and disadvantages

The advantages and disadvantages of epidemiologically based study designs are largely dictated by the context within which they are used. Therefore, advantages and disadvantages will be examined in relation to the type of study questions the technique is used to answer and the method of investigation used to answer them.

Cross-sectional studies document the concurrence of disease and suspected causative factors, both in populations and in individuals or subgroups within populations. For example, Helmert and others (1992) investigated the relationship between social inequalities among those suffering from cardiovascular disease and risk factors in East and West Germany. They found an association between social class and rates of hypertension, hypercholesterolaemia, cigarette-smoking, and obesity. The temptation resulting from surveys such as these to attribute cardiovascular disease outcomes to social inequalities can be very strong. However, in doing so, the disadvantages of the cross-sectional approach are revealed. Measuring potential risk factors and disease outcomes at the same point in time provides information on associations. These associations may or may not be biologically plausible. Where they are, the natural tendency is to infer causation. This may be misleading, because unless one can show a temporal association between cause and effect, one has demonstrated nothing more than biologically plausible association. Such an association is not unimportant, as it may give clues about where, in future prospective studies, limited resources may best be placed in order to demonstrate such temporal relationships.

Therefore, the advantages of epidemiological surveys performed in a cross-sectional manner are that they provide a relatively inexpensive means of determining associations, and of determining whether such associations are statistically significant and have potential biological plausibility. They also allow decisions to be made about where to use research resources in future prospective studies. The disadvantage of such surveys is that they can only infer causation. Unless the researcher is aware of this disadvantage, the potential for misinterpretation is significant.

Epidemiological surveys can also be used retrospectively to examine the link between potential cause and effect. Such studies are known as case-control studies or case-control surveys. The issues surrounding such studies are discussed in greater detail in subsequent chapters, but we will also summarise the major issues here, because the addition of a 'control' group represents a major conceptual leap in the development of public health research techniques, as was shown from a historical perspective in Chapter 1. The addition of a control group (comprising people without the disease of interest) allows comparisons to be made with cases (people with the disease of interest). The technique involves identifying people with the outcome of interest, selecting a group of people similar in most respects (with the exception that they do not have the outcome of interest), and looking back in time to see whether there are differences in exposures to postulated causes. A statistical comparison is then made to determine whether prior exposure is related to the outcomes as currently measured.

It is of critical importance to note that evidence about the prior exposure is also collected in the present day; in other words, the evidence depends on historical records and/or memory of the cases and the controls. You will appreciate that the validity of this technique depends greatly on the accuracy and comprehensiveness of those previous records and/or the memory of participants. It is at this point that significant biases (systematic errors that distort the measured association between exposures and outcomes) can be introduced. For example, if the alleged association has been the subject of speculation in the press, people with the outcome of interest may more readily recall prior exposure, regardless of whether they really had a greater rate of exposure than the controls.

Another source of potential bias is in the selection of controls. It is important that the controls do not differ from the cases in any way that might affect the outcome of interest (other than in not having disease). If they were to differ on the basis, for example, of age, gender, or other attributes that might be related to the outcome, you may introduce spurious associations.

Results may also be biased if the outcome of interest is potentially fatal. Doing a case-control study in these circumstances will mean that your cases will be people in whom the outcome has not yet progressed so far as to cause death, or they will be survivors, and may therefore be inherently different to those people with the outcome who do not survive.

Case-control studies do have significant advantages. Again, they are relatively inexpensive. When a disease or outcome of interests has a long gestation period following potential exposures, anything other than a retrospective study may take decades to produce results. Finally, when the disease or outcome is rare, the performance of a prospective study, such as a cohort study, may require the gathering of an impractically large population sample to begin follow-up. The particular advantage of a case-control study is evident when a specific health question needs to be answered in a limited period of time with limited resources, which is often the case.

The final form of epidemiological survey to be considered in this section is the prospective cohort study. As is implied by the name, a sample is assembled prior to the development of the outcome of interest. Exposure to putative risk factors or other attributes of interest are measured, and follow-up occurs over a period of time. Members of the cohort who develop the outcome of interest are compared, in relation to the factors measured at baseline, with those who do not.

One of the largest and best known of these studies is the Nurses Health Study (Stampfer et al. 1993). The cohort for this study was established in 1976 when 122 000 registered female nurses aged 30–55 years, residing in eleven states in the USA, completed lifestyle and medical history questionnaires sent by mail. Biennial follow-up questionnaires were sent by mail to update information on life events, cardiovascular risk status, cardiovascular disease, and other health-related events. At baseline measurement, all nurses who reported coronary heart disease, stroke, or cancer (other than non-melanotic skin cancer) were excluded. As a result of the exclusion, 117 000 women were available for follow-up, and follow-up continues to the present day. This study has yielded important data on relationships between a large number of risk factors and a large number of disease outcomes, primarily cardiovascular diseases and cancers in middle-aged, middle-class, White American women.

This study reveals the significant advantage of cohort designs: they provide a powerful means of assessing the relationship between a large number of variables measured at baseline (assuming that a large number of variables were measured at baseline) and virtually any outcome that occurs subsequently, provided that the outcome occurs in a sufficient number of people to provide adequate statistical power. Selecting a very large cohort sample virtually assures such statistical power. If a large cohort, as part of a well-conducted study, cannot detect a statistically significant difference, it is worth asking whether any difference of potential public health significance exists at all.

However, the critical reader will appreciate that these very advantages carry with them the seeds of the cohort study's major disadvantages. The first of these is expense. Assembling so large a cohort and measuring over so long a period of time is a very expensive undertaking, and diverts a large amount of resources from other areas. The justification for such a large expenditure of resources must be good. The second disadvantage is that, if the disease outcome is rare, a substantial cohort sample must be assembled. If the outcome of interest develops slowly, a very long-term follow-up is required. There is a further disadvantage to cohort studies: as they are so powerful and move forward in time, it may appear that they are uniquely capable of establishing causation. This is not so. The observers or researchers cannot manipulate the level of exposure experienced by individuals or groups. Therefore, it can not be disproved that the putative cause may merely be very closely correlated with the real cause 'or may even be related to the participant's choice to be exposed' (Detels 1991, p. 26). This means that an association between a putative risk factor and an outcome may occur because those who are likely to develop the disease prefer a particular sort of behaviour, or exposure, and not because the exposure itself causes the disease. For example, let us assume that disease X in its very early stage of development, before it can be diagnosed, leads to a craving for particular sorts of food — let us say chocolate. Performing a cohort study may lead to the spurious conclusion that there is a causative relationship between chocolate-eating and the development of disease X.

Advantages of epidemiological surveys

- Cross-sectional studies are a relatively inexpensive way of determining whether an association worthy of further study is present in a given population.
- Case-control studies improve the ability to make inferences about causation.
- Short of conducting a true experiment, cohort studies are the most likely method to yield valid data about causation.

Disadvantages of epidemiological surveys

- Cross-sectional studies are weak in their ability to determine causative relationships.
- Case-control studies are sensitive to the biasing effects of having to rely on historical or recalled exposure data.
- Cohort studies are relatively expensive, often requiring a long follow-up period before results can be known.

Some practical principles

As has been pointed out, researchers in epidemiological surveys do not control who is exposed or treated. It appears to be fate, for want of a better term, that determines which people become 'cases' and which people remain non-cases or controls in a cohort study. But, in fact, it is not really fate that determines if the onset of a disease or an outcome of interest is related to sun exposure: the exposure bears some causative responsibility. This has important practical implications for researchers performing case-control or cohort studies if they wish to ensure that their results are true and generalisable.

Because researchers do not control, in a random fashion, who is exposed and who is not, it is possible that exposure or 'caseness' is related to some characteristic that is of interest to the researcher, but that, although associated with the outcome of interest, is not its causative factor. For example, it was once commonly believed that breast cancer was more common among well-educated women. Breast cancer was indeed more commonly diagnosed in such women. It was realised that better educated women would be more likely to familiarise themselves with the techniques of breast self-examination and to recognise the need for regular mammography, increasing the chances that cancer would be discovered in such women. It can be seen, therefore, that ensuring comparability between cases and controls requires careful consideration and selection to ensure that extraneous variables do not differ between the groups under study. Any systematic differences between cases and controls that might be related to exposure or outcomes, but which are not causative, may be mistaken for causative factors.

One of the best techniques for controlling such sources of bias lies in the 'matching' of cases and controls. This means that, for each case, one or more controls are selected on the basis that they possess characteristics in common with the case. Matching most commonly occurs for age, sex, ethnic origin, and socio-economic status. There are, in fact, several similar strategies for minimising the risk of bias, and all involve the careful selection of one or more control groups.

The other significant trap in epidemiological surveys lies in assessing exposure after a disease of interest or outcome of interest has occurred. Think about it. When cross-sectional studies have been done that look at the occurrence of heart disease and diet, a curious association often emerges (Gliksman et al. 1994). It is often found that those who have or have had a heart disease generally possess 'better' diet, smoke less, and are more likely to drink only in moderation than are those people without heart disease. This suggests that wine, women and song in excess probably prevent heart disease. The truth of the matter is revealed in prospective studies. On developing heart disease, many people make fundamental changes to their lifestyle, including cigarette-smoking and fat intake. If these characteristics are measured after diagnosis, when the sequence of events is more difficult to establish, it can appear that fat and cigarette smoke are actually good for you. In other words, the presence of the outcome has directly affected the exposure. The other possibilities are that outcome can affect a person's recollection of possible exposures, or that the presence of an outcome can actually affect the measurement or recording of an exposure.

Two ways to preclude such sources of bias are to attempt to use as many sources of information on potential exposures as possible — including a search of the records for any objective measures of exposure taken at the time of such exposure (often found in industrial settings) — and to 'blind' those who gather the data. In other words, those who gather data on exposure should be as unaware as possible of the hypotheses under study and, preferably, of whether the person they are interviewing has the outcome of interest or not.

Principle of using epidemiological surveys
- Cases and controls must be carefully selected to ensure biases are not introduced.
- Association between two variables does not necessarily mean a causative relationship exists between them.
- The more 'prospective' the study (that is, measurement of exposure precedes that of outcomes), the more able it is to examine causation.

The epidemiology of ethics

The primary ethical consideration when performing epidemiologically based surveys is to use the best technique available in relation to the questions being asked. Should your questions involve hypotheses about causation, it would be inappropriate to draw conclusions from study designs that are incapable of addressing causation. Such designs include cross-sectional surveys and retrospective studies such as case-control studies. On the other hand, where a disease is rare, where a disease or outcome takes a very long time to develop, or where the resources do not exist to gather a sufficient number of people at baseline to detect outcomes with adequate statistical power, it would be misleading and unethical to conduct prospective studies.

Cultural and language barriers are also important. A questionnaire or method validated in one culture or language group may not have the same validity if used in other settings. Good ethical practice demands that the methods and study instruments used are culturally appropriate and have been validated for use in the population under study. It is also incumbent on the ethical researcher to ensure that any language or cultural differences between the interviewer and interviewee are minimised. The use of community interpreters may have a role in this.

As you will come to understand better as you read through the rest of the chapters in this book, good ethical practice and good scientific practice go hand in hand. It is the public health researcher's ethical duty to use those techniques best able to answer the question of interest. It is also incumbent upon the researcher to point out any deficiencies or uncertainties resulting from the form of study used. Such practice makes it unlikely that the applicability or the validity of results will be overstated, or that incorrect decisions or even harmful decisions might be made on the basis of the results of epidemiological surveys.

Recommended reading

Detels, R. 1991, 'Epidemiology: The Foundation of Public Health', in W.W. Holland, R. Detels, & G. Knox (eds), *Oxford Textbook of Public Health*, vol. 2, *Methods of Public Health*, 2nd edn, Oxford University Press, Oxford.
An excellent overview.

Fletcher, R.H., Fletcher, S.W., & Wagner, E.H. 1988, *Clinical Epidemiology: The Essentials*, 2nd edn, Williams & Wilkins, Baltimore.

Ganuli, M., Fox, A., Gilby, J., & Belle, S. 1996, 'Characteristics of Rural Homebound Older Adults: A Community-Based Study', *Journal of the American Geriatrics Society*, vol. 44, pp. 363–70.
This is a good example of epidemiology applied to a community setting, as is Goodman et al. below.

Goodman, R. & Graham, P. 1996, 'Psychiatric Problems in Children with Hemiplegia: A Cross-Sectional Epidemiological Survey', *British Medical Journal*, vol. 312, pp. 1065–9.

Hawe, P., Degeling, D., & Hall, J. 1990, *Evaluating Health Promotion: A Health Worker's Guide*, MacLennan & Petty, Sydney.
A step by step guide to applying epidemiological techniques to the evaluation of health promotion activities

Hill, A.B. 1965, 'The Environment and Disease: Association or Causation?' *Proceedings of the Royal Society of Medicine*, vol. 58, pp. 295–300.
This is the paper that launched a thousand publications.

ICAI Group 1996, 'A Prospective Epidemiological Survey of the Natural History of Chronic Critical Leg Ischaemia', *European Journal of Vascular and Endovascular Surgery*, vol. 11, pp. 112–20.

An example of the application of prospective survey techniques in a community setting

Puska, P. 1991, 'Intervention and Experimental Studies', in W.W. Holland, R. Detels, & G. Knox (eds), *Oxford Textbook of Public Health*, vol. 2, *Methods of Public Health*, 2nd edn, Oxford University Press, Oxford, ch. 12.

Essential reading.

Stufflebeam, D.L. & Shinkfield, A.J. 1984, *Systematic Evaluation: A Self-Instructional Guide to Theory and Practice*, Kluwer-Nijhoff Publishing, Boston.

One for the technically minded masochist.

CHAPTER 4

Observational Designs

In the classical observational experiment, a relatively homogeneous group is randomly assigned into two groups: an experimental group and a control group. The experimental group is subjected to an intervention or exposure, while the control (or comparison) group is not. Members in each group may not necessarily know the group to which they belong. Those actually administering the intervention or exposure also may not necessarily know which people belong in which group so that experimenter bias may be avoided. (This is known as a 'double-blind' experiment.) The outcome (or outcomes) of all these deliberations is then measured prospectively (that is, by follow-up procedures).

But for obvious ethical reasons, the 'classical' model of observational experiment cannot be used when the exposure or the act of withholding an intervention is dangerous. So, while experimenting for positive outcomes or testing the credibility of therapeutic claims is fine, this approach is not feasible for anything that might harm the participants. Other observational studies, then, have been designed for just this problem. Sometimes working from existing medical records and sometimes by directly observing people, these observational studies fall into two broad types.

Observational studies of the *exploratory* type examine a chosen morbidity or mortality event and any number of risk factors that may be involved. All of these are analysed for significant correlations to see if any credible relationship can be found between these and any one or more risk factors. This is a kind of 'fishing expedition' to generate hypotheses for further investigation of a more focused kind (Holland et al. 1991).

Most observational studies, however, are of the *explanatory* kind. There are three types of observational studies that purport to explain the relationship between morbidity or mortality and exposure: cross-sectional studies, cohort studies, and case-control studies. This chapter will discuss these particular methods.

Cross-sectional studies aim to measure the prevalence of both disease and risk factors simultaneously, in a once-only physical examination or social encounter with the people in whom they are interested. In cohort studies (also known as prospective studies), the risk factor or exposure is measured and then one or several follow-ups are conducted to see in whom and when the disease appears. This study monitors *future* outcomes of exposure. Finally, the case-control study — also known as the retrospective or trohoc study ('trohoc' is 'cohort' spelt backwards) — the disease is measured first and then the study searches for *past* exposures. Although not necessarily employing randomised controls, cohort and case-control models do use matched or stratified controls. And, of course, there are situations in which a control cannot be randomised.

Some examples

Cross-sectional models

Hill and others (1990) conducted a cross-sectional study of tobacco- and alcohol-use among school students that was designed to assess prevalence of these activities. A total of 351 schools participated in the study. Here, a simple survey is distributed to randomly selected schools. In each school, eighty students were randomly selected across predetermined year levels. The study confirmed the continuing downward trend in smoking among young people, but found that significant numbers are still engaged in these activities. The study is a 'snapshot' of prevalence without the use of controls; it is not an 'experimental design'.

Lewis, Mason, and Srna (1992) studied the carbon monoxide (CO) exposure levels in ninety-eight Australian blast furnace workers: fifty-two CO-exposed workers and forty-six controls from the production areas of the plant. Their sample was stratified by smoking habits. They found that CO levels in the blood were highest for heavy smokers but also, for some non-smokers, the carbon monoxide haemoglobin (COhb) levels approached the safety standard limit.

In both the old Doll and Hill study (1964) and the recent one by Lewis, Mason, and Srna, the researchers conducted their work over a single time period. For Doll and Hill, patients were interviewed only once to obtain the needed data. For Lewis and her colleagues, the research event was spread over three weeks. Expired air samples and venous blood samples were taken from subjects.

However, more than a few observational studies do not interview anyone, relying instead on earlier observational data collected by others. Helsing and Monk (1985), for example, analysed cat and dog ownership among suicides and matched controls to see if there was any material association between pet ownership and suicide. They found none. Nevertheless, these studies well illustrate that observational studies, of any of the three styles described, do not need to make the initial observations themselves. However, what is required is, first, that the clinical observations have been made fairly precisely by someone somewhere and that these records are available, and second, that some arrangement is made to enable the researchers to procure matched or stratified control groups.

Case control

These cases are interesting because they begin with the outcome and then work back from there to search for risk factors or influences that may be responsible for that outcome. These study designs employ matched or stratified controls, and more than a few employ existing medical or administrative records.

The famous early study by Doll and Hill (1950) illustrates rather well the approach taken in this type of work. Employing social workers, Doll and Hill interviewed about 700 people with lung cancer in twenty hospitals around London. An equal number of controls were interviewed about their smoking habits. Comparisons were made between those with lung cancer and those with cancer of the bowel and stomach. Comparisons were also made between these groups and those free of cancer but hospitalised for other conditions. Controls were of the same sex and age group, and from the same hospital. A positive association between smoking and lung cancer was observed.

Dodds and his colleagues (1993) examined congenital abnormalities in children of cancer patients. The records of some 86 000 mothers and fathers of children born with anomalies were matched by the same number of parents whose offspring were born without such anomalies. Fifty-four mothers and sixty-one fathers who were diagnosed, or had been diagnosed with cancer, were identified and matched with controls.

No association could be found between the diagnosis and cancer treatment of parents and subsequent birth of children with congenital abnormalities.

Olsen, Neilsen, and Schulgen (1993) investigated the risk of childhood cancer in those living, or who had lived, near high-voltage facilities. The researchers selected 1701 children newly diagnosed with leukemia, malignant lymphoma, or tumour of the central nervous system, and matched them for sex and date of birth with between two and five controls who lived elsewhere. The parents of the cases and controls were identified through the Danish population register, and the residential history of each child was identified retrospectively. Each address was identified, right down to the street, building number, and side of the building in which these families resided. This information was then checked against a typographic map of existing high-voltage overhead and underground cable. A small association between these magnetic fields and the childhood cancers was identified.

There have been some imaginative case-control studies of morbidity and physical mobility. Thompson and others (1990) studied the effectiveness of bicycle helmets in preventing facial injury. They compared over 200 bicyclists with facial injuries with over 300 others with injuries to other parts of the body. They found that helmets had some protective effect on the upper face, but not on the lower face.

Steenland and others (1990) looked at lung cancer and truck driving in the Teamsters Union. They used retrospective data collected from next of kin and work histories taken from the union. An earlier study by Stein and Jones (1988) examined the involvement of large trucks in crashes. Stein and Jones actually examined crash sites themselves. One week later at each crash site, at the same time of day as the original crash, they selected three trucks for comparison. Truck and driver characteristics were then compared. Double-trailer trucks and single-unit trucks pulling trailers were over-represented in the crashes, regardless of other factors.

Strom and others (1994) interviewed patients diagnosed with systemic lupus erythematosus (SLE) and their age-matched friends to find no relationship between this disease and silicon breast implants. In a similarly interesting study, Bremond and colleagues (1986) interviewed fifty women with breast cancer and 105 controls to discover that cases were more likely than controls to have experienced a 'depleting life event' in the preceding five years, to be committed to external appearances of 'niceness', and to suppress feelings, particularly anger. Professional and salespeople beware!

Cohort or prospective studies

Cohort studies ('cohort' is 'trohoc' spelt backwards!) measure suspected risk factors or exposures and then follow up their respondents some days, weeks, or years later to ascertain whether ill effects have developed. They are seen as more scientific (that is, capable of satisfying more of Hill's criteria).

Westin (1990) employed this approach on eighty-five employees made redundant by a sardine-processing factory and matched these with eighty-seven employees of a 'sister factory', which did not close. The unemployed workers were then interviewed and examined over a ten-year period. Sickness and disability were significant features of the case group.

There are studies of the initial effects of the grounding of an oil tanker near a small community off the coast of Scotland (Campbell et al. 1993); the 'health effects' (the reverse actually) of swimming at certain polluted beaches in Sydney (Corbett et al. 1993); the association between socio-economic disadvantage and child morbidity or developmental delay (Bor et al. 1993; Najman et al. 1992); corneal arcus and the development of coronary heart disease (Chambless et al. 1990); psychosocial work characteristics and cardiovascular disease risk (Greenlund et al. 1995). The usual concerns about smoking and mortality are also represented (Doll et al. 1994a and b) along with some highly interesting studies on subjects such as an examination of breast and ovarian cancer after infertility and *in vitro* fertilisation (Venn et al. 1995). There is even a cohort study investigating the quality of semen in Parisian men during the past twenty years (Auger et al. 1995), which used samples from Parisian semen banks! Truly there are no limits to the public health imagination . . .

Advantages and disadvantages

The diversity of the studies listed above highlights the main advantages of observational studies for the public health researcher. In observations that are cross-sectional, researchers are able to examine the immediate effects of certain exposures, particularly if the effects are acute and dissipate quickly (which they do in the Lewis et al. study of CO exposure in blast furnace workers).

In cohort studies, the public health researcher is less reliant on a respondent's ability to recall distant events or exposures, or on old and incomplete medical records. The researcher is there at the beginning of the exposure and is able to record this in fine detail before beginning the sometimes lengthy task of follow-up. This is a particularly important advantage when details of exposure are not available or are poorly understood, such as is the case with psychosocial work conditions or the physical impact and exposure details of the grounding of an oil tanker on a community in close proximity. And, of course, cohort designs are essential when the details of the exposure are certain but the outcome is not. The evolving effects of a new drug or intervention are good examples of the need for this particular design.

In case-control designs, the observational method has several other advantages. Holland and others (1991) discuss three of these. First, case-control researchers make efficient use of sampling rare diseases. They are able to use the available cases well and select their controls to match. Second, case control permits rapid evaluation of diseases where the time frame between exposure and the development of the disease is long (for example, cancer or cardiovascular disease). Third, unlike

Advantages of observational methods
- They offer flexible design options.
  - **1** They can be exploratory or explanatory.
  - **2** They can search past, immediate, or future exposures and/or outcomes.
  - **3** Rapid or long-term assessment is possible.
  - **4** They can study several risks or exposures or single occurrences
- They can be inexpensive.
- They can provide accurate long-term assessments of early exposures.
- They can identify new or poorly understood outcomes.
- The immediate effects of certain exposures can be identified and assessed.
- They can make efficient use of sampling in the case of rare diseases.

some cohort studies, case-control designs can be inexpensive in terms of time and personnel. Of course, all observational designs have the advantage of being useful as exploratory or explanatory tools for public health research, and this underlines their inherent flexibility as methods in this area.

But there are also problems with observational methods. For instance, Holland and others (1991) outline four limitations of the case-control method. First, case-control methods are not practical for cases of rare exposure. Second, historical information can be difficult to validate. Third, relevant co-factors are difficult to measure or detect. And, finally, the sequence of exposure and disease may be obscured, especially by intervening variables.

More widely applicable in all observational methods is the problem of sample selection, also sometimes referred to as 'caseness'. This problem can be summed up with the question 'What is a "case"?'. For example, when assessing malaria, what will count as a case: someone with proven malarial parasites in the blood? or someone with symptoms consistent with malaria? Who will be included in a study of suicides: those who leave notes to say they have deliberately taken their lives? or simply, among others, all those found dead from domestic poisoning? What tests will determine whether a cancer, or any other disease process, is present in a particular potential subject? These problems of sample selection also apply to the selection of control groups: How many subjects are to be included in the selection? How are they to be 'matched'? What criteria are to be used?

These problems highlight the general problem of bias. As Sackett (1979) and Skrabanek (1993) remind us, observational studies are known to be prone to 'at least 56 different biases'. These different sources of bias range from the problem of false positives and false negatives in diagnostic groups to a diversity of other headaches such as Berkson's paradox (hospital samples may be atypical of the general community); the Neyman fallacy (the survival rate may falsify the impression of incidence, so cases should be selected from newly diag-nosed cases); selective referral; poor subject cooperation; incomplete reporting; and even the refusal to participate at all. (See Holland et al. 1991 for a full discussion of some of these.)

The criteria for 'abnormal' levels of almost anything may be con-tested, or conversely, the boundaries of what others might consider to be 'normal' may lend themselves to charges of 'bias'. In interviews, respondents may have problems of recall, may lie to please or to appear pleasing, or may be led, through poor interview technique or design, to give atypical responses. Records may be dated, incorrect or incomplete. They may even be illegible.

The reliability of much data employed by different observational studies has also been frequently called into question. Flanders and O'Brien (1989) and Feinstein and company (1989) debate the problems and significance of conflating incidence data with prevalence data. Earlier, Feinstein (1979) lamented the overreliance on existing sources of data and the rather disturbing habit of not selecting subjects by physical or diagnostic examination. Too many observational studies look like secondary analysis instead of incorporating the clinical scrutiny that they were designed to include.

Smith and Phillips (1992) — in their own study and in a similar study conducted with their colleague Neaton (Smith, Phillips, & Neaton 1992) — discuss the problems of confounding variables in observational epidemiological work. The independent effects identified by many studies may not be what they seem: they may not be truly independent but, rather, simply associations with yet-to-be-identified 'independent' variables. For example, they remind us that coronary heart disease has 280 'risk factors' — none so great as being alive!

Cervical cancer is commonly thought to be associated with a sexually transmitted agent, but notwithstanding the strong evidence for this, other variables also have 'evidence'. Not eating carrots ('carrot refusal'?), a history of induced abortion, alcohol, the practice of early masturbation, low folate intake, high parity, and cigarette-smoking have all been implicated. Smith, Phillips and Neaton (1992) note that smoking may be a good example of a confounding variable. Smoking is associated with early loss of virginity and multiple partners, and these factors, rather than some tobacco toxin, may lead to some sexually transmissible agent.

Finally, there are debates about the appropriate way to analyse the data when one finally has them all in. The limitations and flaws in certain statistical operations are frequently debated. Some workers argue, for example, that the idea that p-values (statistical levels of significance) have evidential meaning is a mistaken belief. (For an overview of this debate, see Greenland 1989; Woolson & Kleinman 1989; but also Goodman & Royall 1988; Walker 1986; Poole 1987; and Thompson 1987). So what are we to do?

The central idea of reminding readers about the problems behind any single method is not to provide justification for dismissing or downplaying the value of that method. Methods — all methods — continue to be used amid criticism because often their value outweighs their disadvantages. Many of the problems that co-researchers raise as criticisms of any particular method, therefore, can usually be dealt with by applying three pragmatic principles in research: peer review, triangulation, and finally, limitations and explanations.

Ideally, no empirical research should be conducted by a lone researcher, or even by a group that does not consult with other researchers who are not directly involved with the research. There are important gains to be made by consulting colleagues outside the research project. The outsider can often see methodological issues that have been overlooked by a too-involved gaze. This is particularly the case with regard to ethical issues, where a major investment in a project (in time and personnel) may encourage researchers, even unintentionally, to minimise issues of consent or subject comfort. In the same way, outsiders may provide input about caseness that the interested parties may have overlooked. This is particularly important when a project has an important clinical or technical element in which the research team itself does not have an over-abundance of expertise.

Similarly, it is also a good idea to consult with more than one resident data-analyst about possible statistics to use. There are many ways to approach data-analysis, and we can all develop loyalties and habits that, if nothing else, we might usefully justify and explain to ourselves (and, in print, others) from time to time. Statistics is a discipline that is constantly changing, and opinions about the best way of doing things can change. A project can benefit when researchers keep abreast of any such changes.

The question of bias can also be usefully addressed by disinterested parties, and any biases that are identified can be corrected. If it is impossible to correct a bias, team members or outside parties may develop arguments or research design modifications to minimise its influence. A problem encountered for the first time might usefully be laid at the door of a colleague who is known to have more experience with that problem, as he or she may have a suggestion for dealing with it. It is better to receive comments such as these during the research process than after publication!

The principle of triangulation is the rather simple idea of combining methods. In observational studies, it is common for the design to include the combination of, for example, clinical interviews and a search of existing records. Most interestingly, however, each of these methods tends to apply to different stages of the research design rather than acting as cross-checks of the same stages.

For example, one may perform clinical interviews with respondents concerning certain exposures, as did Lewis and her colleagues with CO exposures in smokers and non-smokers at a blast furnace plant (1992), but one may also conduct physical examinations. Lewis and colleagues, when testing before and after CO exposure, were forced to reclassify two 'non-smokers' into their smokers category because venous blood samples taken before CO exposure showed mild CO elevation consistent with other smokers in their study.

All too rarely, clinical interviews are cross-checked by use of existing records or observations. All too often, existing records could have been cross-checked by interviewing or physical examination of subjects, but were not. Often this procedure might have led to more time and expense, but it also might have led to a stronger and more confidant, and perhaps more credible, set of conclusions.

Finally, few studies are perfect, and it is therefore imperative, when publishing our findings, to discuss not only the project's limitations but also the case for the use of one set of methods, statistical operations, or sample instead of other alternatives. As consumers, reviewers, and producers of public health research, it is essential that we come to expect a high standard of pragmatism in the presentation of results. The approach and design of a study always call for explanation, because no research occurs in an academic vacuum; it is carried out in a sea of diverse and contested positions about the 'best way' to do things. With these points in mind, how might we approach observational studies?

Some practical principles

One of the most important principles to apply to all observational studies, whatever their particular approaches, is first to decide whether the study will be for exploratory or explanatory purposes. Feinstein (1988) argues that 'fishing' exercises through different data sets — what he terms 'data dredging' — is poor science. But, just as dredging increases the depth of a lake, this method may deepen our understanding of data, and occasionally turn up unexpected and useful surprises for the researcher with a keen and sensitive eye. If, however, you wish to identify a particular association, then you are indeed beholden to develop specific hypotheses to test that hunch clearly and specifically.

After this first decision, it is important to develop strict and well-defined criteria for sample selection. What criteria will be used for inclusion and what criteria for exclusion? What measures have been taken to eliminate false positives and negatives? How will exposure be defined and measured? These questions lead to broader questions of bias, and Cole (1979: 25) suggests developing a list or catalogue of possible biases and the methods undertaken to control them.

To begin observational work you will need to:
- decide on an exploratory or explanatory approach
- develop criteria for sample selection
- develop a list of possible biases and strategies to minimise these.

For case-control studies, you should first define the disease state and then locate the cases or individuals at risk. The controls should then be chosen with a careful eye to what matching criteria are used (taking account of age, race, neighbourhood, gender, and so on). The sources of exposure information then need to be identified: self reports, medical or occupational records, serological markers and so on. Holland and others (1991) recommend the importance of identifying not only the presence of the exposure but also, of course, the intensity and duration.

So for case controls you will need to:
- define the disease state, and matching criteria for controls
- locate cases and match with controls
- identify sources of exposure information.

For cohort studies, one may focus on sections of the general public in which there is a heterogeneity of exposure or perhaps a particular exposed group or group with a special lifestyle of interest. The earlier comments about sample selection of cases and controls apply equally here. Choose and match carefully with clear and precise operating criteria.

At this point, some baseline measure or estimate of health must be established from existing sources, interviews, or clinical or physical examination. Sometimes it may also be important to include environmental factors in this initial assessment: air pollution levels, dietary intake, average daily hours of sunlight, and so on. In connection to this, one must also remember to be cognisant of confounding variables. Wherever possible, co-variables or related risks should be identified and included so that these can be factored into any subsequent analysis. Establish the basis for follow-up next: how, when, and where respondents will be needed again.

For cohort studies, you will need to:
- define and delimit criteria for exposure
- identify a special group or lifestyle at risk, or a population in which exposure is variable within the group
- choose cases and controls using clear criteria
- establish a baseline of health and environment (if relevant)
- identify and include co-variables in data-collection
- establish the basis for follow-up with respondents.

Observing ethics

The ethical requirements of observational studies are all the usual ones, except that not only might one apply these to subjects and respondents, but also in the use of existing records. These ethics may be described as attention to informed consent, confidentiality, safety, and the avoidance of cheating and of the negative uses of research.

Consent should be informed consent and not simply a request that people participate. They should be given a brief but clear explanation of the research, its aims, procedures, and the possible benefits and risks to them and/or the wider community. In some cases, if next of kin are to be involved, consent might need to be obtained from the institution or medical practice responsible for managing the case. Heuser and others (1988) found that, although the vast majority of next of kin did not mind being contacted, some of them did.

The issue of consent should also extend to the examination and use of existing records and other people's data. Consent will always need to be sought to use the medical records or data archives of government or private research institutes. And remember that permission to use data may not necessarily extend to permission to publish it, so that this issue also needs to be clarified or cleared with owners of data.

This brings us to other issues about confidentiality. Obviously it is important that participants are not identified and that private or identifying information be kept strictly within the research group. There are no criteria for determining which information is 'private' enough for consideration. All patient information that can be identifying should be protected in this way.

There are other issues that might be included in any consideration of confidentiality in observational designs. If one is using a cohort study, for example, to study exposure of certain foods or work practices or chemical exposures, one must be careful not to identify brands or premises when reporting results. Unless the results are highly significant, even the short-term impact of the publication of negative results may have negative effects that may be worse than the original health risk. The avoidance by consumers of a brand can quickly bankrupt a company, or lead to lower sales or the laying off of staff to accommodate poor financial performance. Sometimes it may not be possible to avoid the association of a particular exposure or practice with particular products or companies, but the ethical injunction to consider the implications of your published results for the people employed in those places remains nonetheless.

Considering the safety of people, then, is also not simply a matter of ensuring that your examination procedures do little harm; it is also important that the publication of your results runs the same minimal risk for others. Tests and physical examinations for exposure should be minimal and performed with the subjects' comfort and safety in mind.

It is also worth mentioning that research ethics do not simply entail worrying about the welfare of subjects or respondents. There are ethical issues concerning the conduct of research that apply simply to being a researcher. One should not cheat with any data, or falsify either data sets or results. Neither subjects nor colleagues should be the object of any deception, and this is worth mentioning because cheating continues in all research forums every year. Deception in any research is unethical. In health research, it may also be criminal: it could kill.

Finally, the negative uses or implications of research must be considered. Often results are negative — that is, no interesting effects are observed. This will often lead to a decision not to publish. However, the non-publishing of negative results can lead to a 'file drawer' problem for later researchers in, for example, meta-analysis. Results that are negative, then, might usefully be sent to data registries or archives for storage or registration for future researchers. Alternatively a short letter to an indexed peer review journal can alert others to both the study and its negative result. An associated consideration is the publication of results without warnings or qualifiers. This can cause significant problems if a new association is identified by your study. Heightening this problem is the risk that others (or even yourself) will advise patients to alter their lifestyles on the basis of one study. As M. Angell (1990) warns, there is little value in such 'knee jerk' advice because of the high risk of error. Unless the risk is large, makes obvious sense, or the change is not onerous, changes should not be recommended. Further studies and strong associations need to appear in the literature before action is taken, otherwise every publication of a public health study will (as indeed they sometimes do) lead to widespread community paranoia and hypochondriasis.

Recommended reading

Dwyer, J.H., Feinleib, M., Lippert, P., & Hoffmeister, H. (eds) 1992, *Statistical Models for Longitudinal Studies of Health*, Oxford University Press, New York.

This book is for the statistically curious reader.

Feinstein, A. 1988, 'Scientific Standards in Epidemiologic Studies of the Menace of Daily Life', *Science*, vol. 242, 2 December, pp. 1257–63.

This provides a critical but thought provoking assessment of these designs.

Holland, W.W., Detels, R., Knox, G., et al. 1991, *Oxford Textbook of Public Health*, vol. 2, *Methods of Public Health*, 2nd edn, Oxford University Press, Oxford.

More in-depth discussion of these methods is provided by this text.

Journal of Chronic Diseases 1979, special issue, vol. 32, nos 1 & 2.

Devoted to debating appropriate methodologies for case-control studies, this special issue will be of interest to the statistically curious reader.

Kelsey, J.L., Thompson, W.D., & Evans, A.S. 1986, *Methods in Observational Epidemiology*, Oxford University Press, Oxford.

Again this book provides more in-depth discussion of these methods.

Woolsen, R.F. & Kleinman, J.C. 1989, 'Perspectives on Statistical Significance Testing', *Annual Review of Public Health*, vol. 10, pp. 423–40.

Again, this is for the statistically curious reader.

The next three references are general guides to epidemiology that have excellent chapters on observational designs:

Hennekens, C.H., Buring, J.E. 1987, *Epidemiology in Medicine*, ed. S.L. Mayrent, Little Brown & Co., Boston, especially chapters 5–8.

Rothman, K.J. 1986, *Modern Epidemiology*, Little Brown & Co., Boston.

Schlesselman, J.J. 1982, *Case-Control Studies: Designs, Conduct, Analysis*, Oxford University Press, New York.

CHAPTER 5

Randomised Control Trials

The definition of 'randomised control trials' is contained within these three words. It is 'randomised' because participants are allocated to the various study groups in a random fashion. The crux of randomisation is that each participant should, by the process of randomisation, have an equal chance of being placed in any of the groups that make up the study as a whole. The process is analogous to the flipping of a coin. A high-tech version of this — random number generation — is sometimes used to assign people selected to participate in a randomised control trial into one group or another. In public health or medical circles, the group often comprises a treatment group and a control group. The treatment group may receive an intervention for which comparative information is sought. The comparison or control group either receives a standard treatment or, if ethically feasible, no treatment at all. At the end of the trial period, comparisons may then be made between the effects of treatment and of no treatment or alternate treatment on two or more randomised groups.

This type of study is 'controlled' because, as pointed out above, a comparison or control group is used to compare the effect of a particular treatment against another particular treatment or no treatment at all. In all other respects, the two groups should be treated in the same way if valid conclusions are to be drawn about the effect of various treatments or other interventions. During the trial process, the course of both groups is observed and measured, and any differences in outcome, if the test is conducted properly, may then be attributed to that intervention.

The study can be regarded as a 'trial' because a randomised control trial is a special type of cohort design in which many, if not all, the aspects of the study are determined by the investigators. The type of intervention, the settings in which intervention is conducted, and the length of intervention are all under the control of the trial coordinator or research team. In a properly designed randomised control trial — unlike case-control studies (in which exposure to putative agents are not under the researchers' control) or cohort studies (in which people essentially help select various groups by virtue of their behaviours or preferences) — these aspects are under the control of the researcher.

In effect, the researchers are conducting an experiment (a trial) that is in many ways akin to experiments conducted in a laboratory setting. The process of randomisation and the use of a control group, or of a control-comparison design, make it possible, to a far greater degree than with any other study, to hold constant all factors that may determine outcome — apart from the treatment/control factor being manipulated by the researchers of course.

Potentially, such a study can yield very powerful results with regard to inferring causation. If randomisation has been effective, all variables (other than the one under active study) should be randomly and roughly equally distributed over all treatment groups. Therefore, the only variable that could account for differences between the two groups at the end of the study, compared with any differences in the two groups at the beginning of the study, may be reasonably attributed to the variable manipulated by the researchers. As a randomised control trial is also prospective, it meets many of the criteria referred to in chapter 3 and included in Hill's tests of causality.

But before you get carried away (perhaps to participate in a randomised control trial), you should be aware that there are, arguably, two worlds: the ideal world of the experimenter and the world we actually inhabit, otherwise known as 'the real world'. If randomised control trials are so powerful (and indeed they are), why are they not used to a greater extent? These are issues we will explore in this chapter by reference to specific examples and ethical considerations. By the end you should have a better appreciation of why the world of ideas, as envisioned by Plato, can rarely be achieved in the world of forms that we inhabit.

Some examples

Dwyer and others (1979) were interested in whether physical activity could affect coronary heart disease risk factors in primary- (elementary) aged school children. In order to assess the effect of physical activity on coronary heart disease risk factors, they devised a randomised control trial of the effects of two different physical activity programs on coronary heart disease risk factors, on academic performance, and on classroom behaviour. The subjects were 500 children (with a mean age of ten years) in South Australia.

During the fourteen-week intervention period, children were involved in an endurance fitness program or a skills program, or else they participated as controls. The fitness group spent fifteen minutes in the morning and one hour in the afternoon every school day engaged in organised physical activity. The emphasis was on endurance exercises. A second activity group focused on particular activities that improved various perceptual motor skills, such as catching and throwing a ball or non-strenuous dancing and other non-aerobic exercises. The control group continued with its usual school program, which included only three half-hour periods of organised physical activity per school week, little of which was said to be of the endurance kind. The results showed that the fitness group experienced significant gains in physical-work capacity (a measure of cardiovascular fitness) and decreases in body fat compared with both other groups. Changes in a number of coronary heart disease risk factors, including systolic blood pressure and plasma lipids, did not differ between the groups. Interestingly, both the fitness and skill groups demonstrated improvements in classroom behaviour compared with the control group, although no differences in academic performance were observed.

The effect of fish oil supplements on blood pressure was examined in a double-blind randomised cross-over trial of fish oil supplementation and cholesterol (Lofgren et al. 1993). Participants, recruited as part of the Minneapolis Veterans Affairs Medical Centre trial on the effects of fish oil and serum cholesterol, were aged under sixty years. Blood pressure was recorded at baseline, and then after a four-week 'lead-in' period, subjects were randomised to receive twelve weeks of safflower oil (control oil) followed by a four-week 'washout' and a second period consisting of twelve weeks of fish oil. Another group experienced the same treatment but in reverse order. The researchers reported no significant changes from pre-treatment values in systolic or diastolic blood pressure with the use of fish oil supplements.

When theories emerged that linked folate deficiency during pregnancy with neural-tube defect in newborns (such as spina bifida), Laurence and colleagues (1981) performed a randomised controlled double-blind trial in South Wales. Before conception, sixty of the women selected agreed to take four milligrams of folic acid a day before and during early pregnancy. Fifty-one women were allocated to placebo treatment. The results showed that there were no recurrences of neural-tube defect among compliant mothers, but there were six in total among those who did not take folic acid. It was concluded that folic acid supplementation was a cheap, safe, and effective method of primary prevention of neural-tube defects, although the researchers recommended that be confirmed in a larger multi-centre trial.

Following the emergence of theories suggesting that vitamin A supplementation may reduce child mortality and morbidity in nutritionally deprived environments, several randomised control trials were instituted to test this hypothesis. Among them was a study on child morbidity and mortality following vitamin A supplementation in Ghana (Ross et al. 1995). In this randomised controlled community trial, a vitamin A supplementation scheme involving 25 939 preschool children was undertaken. The researchers devised two double-blind, randomised, placebo-controlled trials of large doses of vitamin A, administered at intervals of four months in adjacent populations in North Ghana. They found that such vitamin A supplementation significantly reduced the overall incidence of severe illness (especially diarrhoea with dehydration), clinic attendances, hospital admissions, and mortality. Other studies, such as that performed by Sommer and others (1986), which was conducted in 450 villages in Northern Sumatra (Indonesia), have also shown that vitamin A supplementation has a significant beneficial impact on childhood mortality.

Randomised control trials can provide information not just on relatively narrow clinical matters, but also on wider matters of socio-demographic interest. For example, Brooks-Gunn and others (1994) wished to examine whether early educational intervention influences maternal employment, education, fertility, and receipt of public assistance and health insurance in the USA. To assess these effects, a randomised control trial of the efficacy of early education on the outcomes of 985 low-birth-weight, premature children was devised. It was called the Infant Health and Development Programme. In this study the families in eight locations received either paediatric follow-up and referral (known as the 'follow-up group') or paediatric services and early intervention services (known as the 'intervention group') for the first three years of the child's life. Assignment to each group was of a randomised nature. The results showed that mothers in the intervention group were employed for more months and returned to the workforce earlier than those in the follow-up group only. These results provided convincing evidence that providing appropriate support and educational services to families, even though the focus is on the child and parenting behaviour, could have the potential to increase parental employment and increase the efficiency of health and welfare services for those who are not employed.

The unique ability of the randomised control trial design to yield valid data on causation has also been used to assess the effect of different diets on weight loss. Baron and others (1986) conducted a three-month randomised control trial among 135 overweight subjects. Two sets of dietary advice were given. Each provided approximately 1000 calories per day but differed in fibre, carbohydrates, and fat content. Information on weight and eating habits, as well as measures of lipoprotein and glucose metabolism, were obtained at entry, after one month, and again after three months. Even though similar calorific intake was observed, those in the low carbohydrate/low fibre diet group tended to lose more weight than those on higher carbohydrate/higher fibre regimen. This pattern was particularly marked among women and participants under the age of forty. However, only minor differences in serum lipoprotein (blood fats) patterns were noted during the diet period.

In order to assess the effect of iodine deficiency on intellectual capacity, a number of randomised controlled trials were undertaken. The results of these trials showed that iodine deficiency *in utero* and before pregnancy was clearly linked to significant developmental and intellectual impairment (Hetzel 1995). These findings led to widespread supplementation programs in areas where iodine deficiency represented a significant public health problem — such as the European alpine regions, Switzerland, Austria, France, Italy and Germany — as a result of iodine-deficient soils. This was not just a European problem, but was also seen in a number of developing countries such as Papua New Guinea and China. The iodine-deficiency story gives perhaps one of the clearest examples of how randomised controlled trials can lead to major public health programs and benefits for populations as a whole. It is the power of the experimental design, in terms of satisfying Hill's criteria for causality (1965), that can provide clear information and motivation for such large public health undertakings.

Advantages and disadvantages

The randomised control trial has revolutionised the way in which we decide whether a treatment or other intervention will do more harm than good. The prospective nature of this type of study and the randomised distribution of variables (other than the variables of interest) have made the randomised control trial the cornerstone for evidence-based medicine and evidence-based public health interventions.

These research techniques provide valid evidence not only on whether one treatment is better than another on given criteria, but also on the extent to which it is 'better', as well as the circumstances under which it might be better. Even where, for one or more reasons, a properly designed randomised control trial is impossible to carry out, the design can still be used as a point of reference against which to judge the validity of other forms of study. It is partly because of the lack of sufficient randomised control trials in relation to a number of public health issues that there remains some controversy about the value of many everyday clinical treatments and public health interventions.

One of the greatest barriers to the institution of randomised control trials in relation to many research questions is their expense and difficulty. Yet the question of cost versus benefit has been addressed in at least one area. Drummond and others (1992) attempted to assess whether the benefits to society of an investment in randomised controlled trials exceeded the costs of such studies. As an example, they assessed the cost benefit of the Diabetic Retinopathy Study, a major clinical trial funded by the National Eye Institute in the United Kingdom from 1972 to 1981. The estimated cost of the trial was US$10.5 million. The estimated net savings to society as a result of increased knowledge of the causes and prevention of retinopathy was US$2.8 billion, resulting from a gain to the study population of 279 000 vision years. The authors noted that, in order to achieve the full benefit of the results of randomised control trials, strenuous efforts must be made to disseminate the results in order ultimately to change clinical or public health practices. They also made the point that it is the technical advantages of properly conducted randomised control trials that make them more likely than other forms of study to change clinical practice and therefore yield maximum results.

There are, however, many disadvantages to be considered in relation to randomised control trials. In a highly provocative article by J. Herman

(1995), it was argued that the randomised control trial was 'irreversibly dead'. To support this view, Herman cited the results of the Global Utilisation of Streptokinase and Tissue Plasminogen Activator for Occluded Coronary Arteries (GUSTO) study. Despite being technologically advanced, its use of over 40 000 patients and 1000 separate sites in fifteen countries yielded ambiguous results. The large cost of this study and the ambiguity of its outcomes led Herman to conclude that the randomised control trial had simply become too complex, inconclusive, and unethical (we will return to this matter later) to be taken for granted as a 'gold standard'.

Another important disadvantage of a particular sub-group of randomised control trials — the placebo control trial — was highlighted by Aspinall and Goodman (1995). They pointed out that, in a number of studies on effective medications, significant numbers of patients were denied access to existing drugs or to new drugs as a result of placebo designs. This matter will also be further discussed when we consider ethics in relation to randomised control trials.

Further limitations of the randomised control trial were raised in relation to the testing of AIDS vaccines by Mariner (1989). It was Mariner's view that, at the time, so little was known of the human immunodeficiency virus (HIV) that the randomised control trials of two vaccines that were then underway were premature and may eventually lead to unintended consequences. This argument highlights concerns about treating this potentially powerful scientific method as a 'black box' into which hypotheses can be thrown and conclusions drawn from the other end. It was Mariner's contention that, where little is known of the mechanisms underlying supposed therapeutic action, the provision of vaccines may create a conflict between the need for expeditious vaccine development and the need to protect human subjects from unreasonable risks. This question goes to the core of arguments over the benefits and risks of scientific study, particularly with human subjects.

One rarely recognised yet extremely important limitation of the randomised control trial is that, while participants may be randomised to various treatment groups, their selection for inclusion in the study itself is usually not random. People tend to self-select for inclusion of randomised control trials by the very act of their agreement to participate. It is not every person who would agree to place themselves in a situation in which they have but a 50 per cent chance of receiving a 'new' treatment or, in some instances, a 50 per cent chance of receiving no treatment at all. This form of self-selection may lead to study results that are internally valid (in other words, that give real data on whether the different treatments affected the study population differently) but that may not be generalisable to the population with the disease or problem of interest as a whole.

A particular sub-issue of this self-selection process was raised by Meyers and others (1994) when they considered whether intravenous drug-users would be likely to enrol in HIV vaccine trials. They provided convincing arguments to suggest that, in the USA, it would be most difficult to recruit intravenous drug-users into HIV vaccine-efficiency trials. Not having representative samples would run the risk of preventing researchers from drawing conclusions about the efficiency of the vaccine in preventing HIV among those people indulging in non-sexual, high-risk behaviours. Such sampling bias would severely limit the generalisability of any study results, and this could not be overcome by randomisation within the study itself.

Similar concerns were raised in relation to randomised control trials of cancer treatments. Research into participant characteristics conducted by Gotay (1991) showed that non-participation in such trials was strongly influenced by physician and patient variables, which may well affect outcomes. For similar reasons, as noted above in relation to HIV, such biases in patient inclusion strongly limit the generalisability of results beyond the study samples tested.

Advantages of randomised control trials
- The trial is prospective in design; exposure *precedes* the development of the outcome.
- The researcher 'manipulates' the exposure status of study participants.
- This study design is capable of satisfying more of the criteria for establishing causality than any other study design.

Disadvantages of randomised control trials
- They are relatively expensive.
- There are ethical issues involved in providing 'placebo' treatments.
- The tendency for inclusion by self-selection may introduce biases that limit generalisability.

Despite these constraints, it is still true to say that randomised control trials contain within their design the potential to provide the strongest scientific evidence for the effects of specific interventions in medicine and public health.

Some practical principles

Randomisation is one of the best ways of minimising the biases that can occur when members of the study sample are assigned to different study groups. If done properly, the effect of randomisation is to ensure that each member has an equal chance of being placed in any of the groups (for example, treatment group or placebo group). However, it is advisable to check whether randomisation has worked by assessing whether, following randomisation, the groups formed are similar in terms of important sociodemographic factors, such as age, gender, and indicators of health status. If so, there can be an increased level of confidence that randomisation has 'worked' in reducing potential biases.

As has been pointed out, although the process of randomisation tends to control many potential sources of bias, the selection of people to include in the randomised control trial in the first place may carry with it sufficient biases to militate against the generalisability of results. Therefore, a great deal of care must be taken in selecting people for inclusion in such trials. There are no hard and fast rules on this.

If you wish to generalise results to the population from which the sample is drawn, then it stands to reason that the group selected should be as similar to that general population as possible. For example, a study that seeks to answer questions about the effectiveness of a new vaccine for children would be of little use if the study sample were made up of adults. Similarly, a study that seeks to test the effectiveness of a new strategy or treatment aimed at preventing heart disease would not tell us much if the sample studied already suffered from that disease.

Often, however, randomised control trials are used to assess various forms of treatment for people who already have disease. It then becomes incumbent on the researcher to select people with the disease who reflect the wider population of people with the same disease. If the treatment is aimed at preventing disease progress, it would be meaningless to draw the study sample from people in the terminal phase of that illness. However, because funding for research tends to be concentrated in tertiary medical teaching areas, the patients selected for inclusion can often be highly atypical, in either socio-demographic characteristics or in characteristics related to the severity or type of disease. This means that the study results may not be easily applicable to a population of interest to the researcher. It is important to be mindful of these potential limitations when interpreting the results of such studies. There is no substitute for an awareness of any differences in characteristics between the study sample and the population of interest, especially when those differences may influence disease or other important outcomes.

Even when great care has been taken in terms of sampling and randomisation, there is yet another possible source of bias. If researchers are aware of who is receiving what treatment, and are aware of the hypotheses, it is possible that, consciously or unconsciously, their assessment of the effectiveness of intervention may be influenced (or biased) by such knowledge. Similarly, if subjects or patients in the trial are aware of the type of treatment they are receiving, it may affect their self-rated response to treatment. The technique to be employed to prevent this is called 'blinding' (in which the patient or the researcher is unaware of which group the person being studied is in), or 'double-blinding' (in which both are unaware).

Blinding is most important when assessment of outcomes are somewhat subjective, although even so-called 'hard' outcomes can be susceptible to biases. Even something that seems objectively verifiable, such as changes on an electrocardiographic reading, can be interpreted differently by different clinicians. Blinding does not mean poking out the eyes. Quite the contrary: a properly conducted double-blind study is best able to ultimately identify any real association between interventions and outcomes.

Principles of use
- Care is needed in sampling to ensure that participants are representative of the population to which you intend to apply the results.
- Truly random allocation to the various study groups is essential if bias (systematic errors) in the results are to be avoided.
- Double-blinding is necessary if other important sources of bias are to be avoided.

Randomly controlled ethics

It may be apparent to you from the material already presented that randomised control trials present unique ethical problems. For example, such techniques cannot be used to study the cause of disease. If you are not sure why, think about it. Under what circumstances would it be ethical to assign people to receive potentially harmful exposures? Conversely, similar ethical considerations apply to the provision of placebo 'treatment'. If it is unethical to assign subjects to receive a placebo when this delays their access to a drug with known effectiveness, it can also be argued that it is unacceptable to delay effective treatment by testing a new drug that might not only be ineffective but also hazardous. It would therefore be reasonable to suppose that, if there is doubt about the efficacy of a new treatment, exposure of some subjects to placebo in a well-designed and executed clinical trial may not continue to pose ethical dilemmas. This, however, is not a universally held position.

A particular ethical consideration comes into play when children are the subjects of randomised control trials. This was most clearly delineated by Harth and Thong (1995) in a study in which they interviewed sixty-four parents after the completion of a clinical trial involving their children. Their results showed that only a small minority of parents realised that drug trials were designed not only to assess the efficacy of the treatment but the safety of it as well. The parents were of the opinion that drug trials conducted by hospitals posed no or little risk. Moreover, a significant minority of the parents offered the view that strict informed-consent procedures followed in the trial were unnecessary because they would do what the doctor advised. Only one-third of the parents were aware of their rights to withdraw their children unconditionally from the trial at any time for any reason. These findings suggest that there may have been significant attitudinal barriers to parental understanding of the informed-consent process, sufficient to compromise the safety of children who are not in a position to give informed consent themselves.

It therefore seems incumbent upon researchers to be particularly careful about explaining rights, responsibilities, and the technicalities and risks of their research proposal when children are involved, as parents cannot be relied upon to exercise balanced and informed consent in the absence of such information.

Recommended reading

Burrows, R.F. & Burrows, E.A. 1995, 'The Feasibility of a Control Population for a Randomized Control Trial of Seizure Prophylaxis in the Hypertensive Disorders of Pregnancy', *American Journal of Obstetrics and Gynecology*, vol. 173, pp. 929–35.
This article provides an example of the randomised control trial applied to the clinical setting.

Department of Clinical Epidemiology and Biostatistics, McMaster University, Hamilton, Ontario 1981, 'How to Read Clinical Journals V: To Distinguish Useful from Useless or Even Harmful Therapy', *Journal of the Canadian Medical Association*, vol. 124, pp. 1156–62.
This outlines an essential skill and is well worth a read.

Feinstein, A.R. 1985, *Clinical Epidemiology: The Architecture of Clinical Research*, W.B. Saunders, Philadelphia.
Feinstein provides an excellent overview of randomised control trials. Chapter 29 is most relevant.

Friedman, L.M., Furberg, C.D., & De Mets, D.L. 1985, *Fundamentals of Clinical Trials*, 2nd edn, Littleton Wright Inc., Cambridge, Mass.

Hetzel, B. 1995, 'From Papua New Guinea to the United Nations: The Prevention of Mental Defect due to Iodine Deficiency', *Australian Journal of Public Health*, vol. 19, pp. 231–4.
This is likely to become a seminal paper.

Institute of Medicine 1985, *Assessing Medical Technologies*, National Academy Press, Washington DC.
This book discusses the uses and abuses of randomised control trials in medical technology assessment.

Meinert, C.L. 1986, *Clinical Trials: Design, Conduct and Analysis*, Oxford University Press, New York.
This offers a good overview.

Weiss, G.B., Bunce, H., & Hokanson, J.A. 1983, 'Comparing Survival of Responders and Non-responders after Treatment: A Potential Source of Confusion in Interpreting Cancer Clinical Trials', *Controlled Clinical Trials*, vol. 4, pp. 43–52.
This discusses important issues that affect the validity of results from randomised control trials.

CHAPTER 6

Quality-Adjusted Life Years (QALYs) or Utilities

There is often a tendency in medical and public health research to concentrate on easily or well-defined health outcomes, measured, for example, in terms of days of hospital stays or of haemorrhagic (bleeding) complication rates in anticoagulant therapies for acutely blocked coronary arteries (heart attack). It is easy to understand the reasons why this is so. Not least among them is the desire for a measure that follows the basic tenets of scientific measure: objectivity and reproducibility (Koestler 1977).

Defining outcomes according to the researcher's or the clinician's need for what is often termed 'hard' data has significant drawbacks. People's experience of their lives and well-being is essentially, and indeed by definition, subjective. Where the assessment of outcomes is driven solely by the needs of researchers or clinicians, there is a risk that studies will ignore the 'real-life' choices between quality and quantity of life that are often made by people when receiving treatment or making lifestyle decisions. This is the basis of the dilemma: quantity is 'objective' and easily measured and therefore is often what is measured. There is a tendency to define health outcomes solely in such terms. Quality is perceived to be less objective and far harder to measure. Until recently, such measures have tended to be ignored. This is despite the fact that measures of quality may be of more relevance to people.

This is probably seen with the greatest clarity when we consider the effectiveness of treatments for cancers. Outcomes are usually measured in terms of years of survival. What could be more objective (or easier) than that? Yet for the recipients of anti-cancer treatments, it is not likely to be the measure that best captures their perceptions of the relative desirability of different treatments and outcomes (Kellehear 1990). Surgery, chemotherapies, and radiation therapies entail significant side effects. Some can be painful, very unpleasant (involving uncontrollable nausea and vomiting, for instance), or distressing. Some can be lethal in their own right. Sometimes, the gains in survival for highly aggressive treatments are measured only in extra weeks or months of life. If fully informed of the likely benefits and drawbacks, what would most people choose? This 'trade-off' between quality and quantity issues totally eludes capture by so-called objective measures such as mortality.

This brings us to the essential difference between cost-effectiveness analysis and cost-utility analysis. The former compares the incremental cost of a given intervention with its incremental effects on outcomes such as cases found, years of lives saved, or infections prevented. The latter compares the same incremental costs with incremental effects on outcomes, where some measure of perceived change in the quality of life is incorporated into the measure of outcome.

There has been an increasing realisation of the importance of social, psychological and emotional factors in people's perceptions of well-being, and of how these influence people's preferences and decisions. This has fuelled the growth in a more complex, holistic approach to assessing the relative values of different health outcomes. These measures have at their core the hypothesis that fully informed people would be willing to make a trade-off between prolonging life and improving the quality of remaining life. These measures are most commonly referred to as quality-adjusted life years or QALYs. They represent a synthesis of mortality probabilities and an assessment of perceived well-being during a given period of time in defined circumstances.

The generation of a QALY involves several important steps. The first is the definition of two or more mutually exclusive health states, relevant to the disease or illness under study. The choice may be as simple as (for example) two years of life with severe angina or one year with no pain, or it may be considerably more complex. The closer the choices reflect those realistically encountered by people faced with treatment choices, the more valid the conclusions are likely to be.

A critical step lies in the development of a scale of preferences for each choice. Generally, the scale assigns a value of 1 for a status of 'full health', with a value of 0 for death. In between these extremes, different scaling values must be enumerated for differing outcomes. There are several methods for determining such a scale, but most involve some form of focused interview to quantify the preferences of a (hopefully) representative sample of people. Two of the more common methods used are the standard gamble and the time trade-off (Drummond 1991).

The standard gamble offers the sample two outcomes: one a treatment with possible results (either death or a return to normal health for the remainder of their lives); the other the certainty of remaining in the 'diseased' or distressed state for the rest of their lives. The probability of a 'successful' treatment outcome can be varied until members of the sample express no preference between attempting treatment or remaining in their current state. The probability setting at which this happens can be used to calculate a preference value for the health state.

The time trade-off approach asks people what amounts of time they would be willing to spend in various health states. For example, a person could be asked to choose between a short remainder of life in good health or a longer period of time in a state of lesser health. The period of time a person is willing to 'trade' can be used to generate a preference value for a given outcome or health state.

You can appreciate (as have many researchers) that there are many alternative ways to devise utility measures to be used in generating QALYs. These have been well summarised elsewhere (Nord 1992). All have their particular advantages and disadvantages.

When the scaling score has been devised, it is then possible to apply it to certain outcomes. A year of life in a state of full health rates a 1. A year of life in a state of health scaled at 0.75 scores a QALY of 0.75. Six months of life in a state of full health scores a QALY of 0.5, and so on.

Opit (1991) has highlighted a number of major problems with the concept of QALYs. QALYs are most often used as a means of resource rationing, and so it is important to recognise and address these problems when they are used. Among them is the limitation inherent in utilising a measure of average collective preferences to quantify a measure of individual utility or preference. Further, there is clear evidence that preferences are not stable over time, age, gender, or changing social and economic contexts. These concerns are magnified when QALYs are combined with cost data to form the basis of resource-allocation. Unless great confidence can be sustained in the philosophical and methodological assumptions underlying the generation of QALYs, the objectivity and validity of the decisions reached may be lower than believed or desired.

Some examples

One of the earliest applications of quality-adjusted life years analysis to clinical decision-making can be found in a study that sought to determine whether the number of coronary artery bypass graft operations funded under the United Kingdom's National Health Service should be increased, decreased, or remain at then present levels (Williams 1985). Were limited resources best directed towards this procedure, or would more QALYs accrue to patients if other contenders for funding received relatively greater priority? Using an early form of interview-based preferred status ratings, which could not be fully categorised as either a 'standard gamble' or 'time trade-off', coupled with data on the effectiveness of different procedures and their relative treatment failure rates, this study was able to show that coronary bypass grafting offered better 'value for money' than other treatments for severe angina or multiple coronary vessel disease. Benefits were calculated in terms of QALYs gained compared with costs incurred for a variety of treatments for several other conditions. This yielded the conclusions that the funding of hip replacement, aortic valve replacement, coronary artery bypass grafting, and the insertion of pacemakers to treat heart block should take priority over funding additional facilities for kidney dialysis and coronary artery bypass grafting for mild angina. The study concluded that the latter procedures incurred higher costs per QALY gained than did the former procedures.

Busschbach and others (1993) sought to discover whether the value placed on health differed at different stages of life. Thirty tertiary-level students and a similar number of elderly people rated the quality of life of hypothetical patients of differing ages who were suffering from end-stage renal disease. By manipulating the time these 'patients' had to wait for transplantation, the utility afforded to health by the two separate age-grouped subjects could be compared. Both groups ranked the utility of health in remarkably similar ways, suggesting the value afforded health was durable throughout life.

The health and economic effects of aerobic exercise in preventing coronary heart disease was examined in a study that costed exercise (jogging), estimated resulting reductions in the rate of coronary heart disease, and assessed the effectiveness in terms of quality-adjusted life years gained (Hatziandreu et al. 1988). The researchers estimated from pre-existing epidemiologic data that 35-year-old male non-exercisers had a lifetime relative risk of coronary heart disease twice that of regular exercisers. The direct and indirect costs associated with exercise, injury, and coronary heart disease were calculated. The results indicated that the economic cost per QALY gained from regular aerobic exercise compared favourably with other preventive or therapeutic interventions aimed at reducing the incidence of coronary heart disease.

A comprehensive literature review compared the cost-effectiveness of various interventions aimed at the prevention and treatment of coronary heart disease (Crowley et al. 1995). Several particularly interesting conclusions emerged. Health promotion and secondary prevention programs were not necessarily the most cost-effective interventions per QALY gained. In some instances, relatively high technology and/or expensive treatments were more cost-effective. An example given involved the use of beta-blocker drugs after acute myocardial infarction (a heart attack), in which the cost per QALY gained was highly favourable. This analysis highlighted the need to consider outcomes as well as costs when deciding where to expend limited resources. Of equal if not greater importance, it underlined the relevance of quality-of-life issues in deciding between the relative desirability of differing outcomes that do not include death.

The quality-of-life issues inherent in the side effects of treatment and in alternative outcomes were considered to make mammographic screening an ideal candidate for cost-utility analysis (Hall et al. 1992). In this study, descriptions of quality of life for women with breast cancer were developed from surveys of women with breast cancer as well as women without breast cancer. The time trade-off technique was then used to derive values for outcomes in breast cancer treatment. The costs of mammographic screening were estimated, including the costs of further investigations and treatment of subsequently confirmed cases. After all this effort, the results on the cost utility of mammographic screening were inconclusive.

Daly and others (1993) sought to measure the impact of menopausal symptoms on women by utilising a measure of the change in their perceived quality of life. Sixty-three women aged 45–60 years were interviewed at a specialist menopause clinic and two general practices in Oxford. Two different methods were used to quantify quality-of-life measurements: a time trade-off and a rating scale. The women gave relatively low QALY ratings to a state of health compromised by significant menopausal symptoms. Comparison of QALY ratings before and after hormone-replacement therapy showed significant improvements, suggesting that such forms of treatment may significantly enhance the quality of life experienced by women during the menopause and in the early post-menopausal period.

A cost-effectiveness analysis of hormone-replacement therapy and lifestyle interventions in the prevention of hip fracture used QALYs as an integral part of the analysis (Geelhoed et al. 1994). The cost-effectiveness of several interventions to prevent osteoporosis was estimated using a decision analytic model for a hypothetical cohort of 100 000 healthy perimenopausal women. Four interventions were analysed: oestrogen from age fifty years for life; oestrogen from age fifty years for fifteen years; oestrogen from age sixty-five years for life; and a lifestyle regime of calcium supplements and exercise. The four interventions were compared with no intervention by contrasting medical and nursing-home costs, life years gained, QALYs gained, and costs per QALY gained. Somewhat surprisingly, the lifestyle intervention proved to be the most expensive in terms of costs per QALY gained, with oestrogen from the age of sixty-five being the most cost-effective of all, suggesting that medical treatment commencing at a later age may offer the best use of limited resources when quality- as well as quantity-of-life issues are factored into the cost-effectiveness equation.

A hypothetical birth cohort of 250 000 non-Aboriginal Australian children was used to determine the cost-effectiveness of different immunisation strategies in the prevention of haemophilus influenzae type b (Hib) disease (McIntyre et al. 1994). The estimates suggested that one dose given at eighteen months of age was the most cost-effective in terms of resulting improvements in QALYs, even though this would result in more deaths than if three doses were given commencing at six months of age. If immunisation schedules were to be determined on solely cost-effectiveness criteria, one cannot help wondering what the QALY rating for parents who lose a child to Hib before eighteen months of age would be.

However, the application of a cost-effectiveness analysis to determine the value of road-safety education in Australia graphically illustrates the potential benefits of this approach (Shiell & Smith 1993). Using a QALYs-saved method, these researchers were able to demonstrate that a moderately effective road-safety education program could yield greater benefits per dollar spent than many medical interventions, including pacemaker implantation, coronary artery bypass grafting, or kidney transplantation. This is food for thought when it comes to deciding on the relative merits of extra funding for health care or for other areas of public expenditure.

Advantages and disadvantages

In the provision of health services and in funding public health initiatives, decisions regarding priorities for resource-allocation are often made on the basis of incomplete data. Even worse is the all-too-common situation in which decisions reflect political expediencies or the need to silence the 'squeaky wheel' — just like in the rest of the economy! However, if decisions are to be made on the basis of equity, they must be driven by outcomes. Outcomes can be measured in terms of health states achieved for given expenditures; comparisons can then be made of outcomes in different areas of intervention; and decisions can be reached about the comparative cost-effectiveness of those interventions.

The most common measures used to assess the effectiveness of various interventions are outcomes such as changes in health status, mortality rates, or other indicators of disease such as blood pressure or national cholesterol profiles. Such measures are relatively easy to obtain and compare, but they tell us little of the *value* of a given outcome to individuals and groups. A measure that combines the utility value of a health state with life expectancy has the considerable advantage of enabling comparisons of qualitative as well as quantitative outcomes. Quality-adjusted life years allow the output of health-care interventions to be compared on the basis of the contribution they make to improvements (or otherwise) in both the *quality as well as quantity* of life.

However, the potential disadvantages can be as great as the potential advantages. The outcome scenarios used to generate QALYs are usually hypothetical constructs. People are asked to *imagine* they are experiencing various potential health states and to indicate their relative preferences for each one. Would they make the same choice if the choice were real? The validity of the utility measure depends in large part on the realism of the hypothetical scenarios used. Depending on how the hypothetical scenarios are constructed, significantly different (and significantly misleading) utility values can result. Therefore, the hypothetical scenarios should be as similar to 'real-life' situations facing real patients as is practicable.

To ameliorate this potential problem, some researchers use 'real' patients as the sample from which to generate utility measures. The disadvantage is that this restricts the utility measurement to one health state per patient. Asking a patient to rate comparative health states for any condition other than the one from which they suffer is arguably no more valid than asking any other member of the public to do the same.

Others have used health professionals such as doctors to provide ratings of comparative health-utility states. The advantage is that health professionals are familiar with the various hypothetical states. The obvious disadvantage is that 'advanced' knowledge may lead to the assignment of comparative values that are fundamentally different from what would be chosen by people with a less extensive knowledge of those conditions (such as patients). Furthermore, health professionals differ from most other members of the general population in terms of factors (such as age and socioeconomic well-being) that may have a direct bearing on the way in which various health states are valued.

Advantages of QALYs
- Used well, QALYs can enhance the equity of outcomes in decision-making.
- QALYs allow decisions about resource-allocations to take quality as well as quantity issues into account.

Disadvantages of QALYs
- Used poorly, QALYs can exacerbate inequities in resource-allocation and outcomes.
- Unless hypothetical scenarios are carefully constructed, the results may be misleading.
- Unless the sample used to generate QALYs is as similar as possible to those to whom the results are to be applied, misleading conclusions are likely.

A further and substantial potential disadvantage is that the strict application of funding according to relative QALY values might mean that some groups in society — for example the elderly, whose treatment is relatively costly per QALY gained — might receive little or no care. This result is the antithesis of the main argument in favour of the use of QALYs — the enabling of equitable resource-allocation (Drummond 1991).

Finally, current cost-per-QALY estimates are valid only (if at all) for interventions at the contemporary stage of treatment methods and knowledge. As treatment techniques improve or change, so too may their true relative values in terms of cost per QALY gained. Therefore, cost and QALY estimates must be updated to keep up with technological and other relevant changes.

Some practical principles

When the quality of life experienced by people is a result of an individual or group intervention, the use of a valid measure of cost-utility should be contemplated. This is especially so when quality of life is the only outcome of importance, as in the treatment of illnesses that do not have death as a possible outcome, such as ringworm or arthritis.

Think about the things people are likely to value in their lives. Think about what is of value in your life — the things that make life worth living. In assessing what makes it all worthwhile, most people would nominate things other than, or as well as, the number of years of life left to them. Health, happiness, the love of friends and family, and the respect of colleagues are some of the things people 'live for'. If you think that these are not of legitimate concern in public health planning and resource-allocation, think again.

To someone facing chemotherapy for cancer, quality-of-life issues loom large. If one form of therapy prolongs life more than another form, but at the cost of a greater degree of nausea and fatigue, which is the preferred form of treatment? Is the value of prolonging years of life, at the cost of some attenuation of the capacity to live that life to the full, the same for all age groups? Or do older people value life differently than younger people?

If limited resources must be divided among a number of competing areas in public health, particularly where none of them have clear-cut cost and mortality/morbidity advantages or disadvantages, careful analysis is required to detect *marginal* differences between programs.

Conversely, cost-utility analysis using QALYs should be avoided where only intermediate output-effectiveness data can be obtained (Drummond et al. 1991). The example used by Drummond and others concerns measured changes in blood pressure, a risk factor for several cardiovascular diseases. In itself, raised blood pressure is asymptomatic and therefore, by definition, cannot measurably affect quality of life until it causes an end-stage disease such as stroke or heart attack. This is an important point to remember, as the misuse of cost-utility analysis can lead to an inappropriate or ineffective reallocation of resources when used by those without a good grasp of the principles underlying the validity of such measures.

Also of critical importance is the necessity of ensuring that the utility values used to generate QALYs are valid. To do this, several basic criteria must be met. We have already discussed some of these, but they are so important that they bear repetition.

The subjects chosen to generate the measures of utility of given health states should be as similar as possible to those to whom you wish to generalise the results. If the results are to be extrapolated to young people, young people should be used to generate those measures. If the results are to be extrapolated to people suffering a terminal illness, then, as far as practicable, people suffering from that type of illness should be used to generate the utility value.

The descriptions of the health states you wish to have evaluated should be as realistic as possible, yet must be presented in a balanced and neutral way. If the language or presentation of the scenario used carries with it, intentionally or otherwise, some bias to suggest a predetermined preferred state, that bias will be reflected in the utility values generated for the different health states presented.

Principles
- To generate QALYs, select a sample that is truly representative of the population to which you intend to apply the results.
- Select the method you wish to use to generate QALYs, and be aware of the assumptions and limitations of each method.
- Use realistic scenarios to generate QALYs.
- Do not contemplate using QALYs where only intermediate output data is available.

Finally, the scenarios and measurements should be capable of producing similar results in separate measurement periods. In other words, your measurement instrument should be reliable (consistent) in its rating results over time (Elvik 1995). Ideally, during the development of your measurement instrument, you should be able to demonstrate this capability by doing multiple measurements over a period of time, both with the same sample and with differing samples. Easy, isn't it?

Ethical qualities

When one cuts through the technical minutiae, the methodological intricacies, and the practical problems in application, what lies at the core is the realisation that QALYs are ultimately about rationing and cost-containment (La Puma 1992). The application of QALYs to policy decision-making will have considerable ethical implications if equity in outcomes is compromised in comparison to other methods of decision-making.

As we have seen, QALYs make a number of questionable ethical assumptions. The method assumes that comparative quality-of-life implications for given outcomes can be measured accurately enough to be used in determining resource-allocation. It also assumes that a utilitarian approach (defined as the greatest good for the greatest number) is the most ethical way of determining the allocation of limited resources. It further assumes that older and sicker patients have less potential to benefit from resources allocated to them than those who are younger and healthier. How do these assumptions measure up?

A cross-sectional survey of Australians revealed a strong preference for the maintenance of egalitarian outcomes in health-care decision-making (Nord et al. 1995). A policy of health utility maximisation received very limited support when the consequence was a loss of equity or a loss of access to services for the elderly or for people with limited potential for improving their health. Time trade-off techniques can be a particular problem in this context. A twenty-year-old is likely to regard three years of life very differently from a seventy-year-old. Too often, QALYs generated for one age grouping are assumed to apply to all age groupings.

QALY measurements project group preferences onto the preferences of individual patients, yet the two are not equivalent. The concept that the preferences of others (sometimes *healthy* others) can be applied to individual patients represents a potential breach of accepted medical and clinical ethics. There is a dynamic tension between efficiency issues in the allocation of resources and clinical ethics when applied at an individual level. The ethical practice of cost-utility analysis depends largely on how these tensions are balanced and resolved. There is a real risk that the limitations of QALYs will be disregarded by politicians and bureaucrats who are impressed by QALYs' ability to generate apparently 'hard' data with which to inform policy decision-making. The risk is that factors of equal or greater importance, such as equity, may be devalued.

The ethical challenge is to come to a sound understanding of what society and individual patients value about health care: 'It is clearly naive to assume that patients wish to maximise quality-adjusted life expectancy. But what do they wish to maximise? The more we learn about this question, the more [ethically] acceptable will be the prescriptive models that seek to guide allocations of medical resources' (Weinstein 1986: 214).

Recommended reading

Drummond, M. 1991, 'Output Measurement for Resource Allocation Decisions in Health Care', in A. McGuire, P. Fenn, & K. Mayhew (eds), *Providing Health Care: The Economics of Alternative Systems of Finance and Delivery*, Oxford University Press, Oxford.

Drummond, M.F., Stoddart, G.L., & Torrance, G.W. 1991, *Methods for the Economic Evaluation of Health Care Programmes*, Oxford University Press, Oxford.

Both works by Drummond should be regarded as essential reading for those who wish to pursue further study in this area

Fallowfield, L. 1990, *The Quality of Life: The Missing Measurement in Health Care*, Condor, London.

The title says it all.

Koestler, A. 1977, *The Act of Creation*, Picador, Ardsley, NY.

Although this is intellectually challenging, it has nothing to do with QALYs. Read it for your general scientific education.

Nord, E. 1996, 'Health Status Index Models for Use in Resource Allocation Decisions: A Critical Review in the Light of Observed Preferences for Social Choice', *International Journal for the Technological Assessment of Health Care*, vol. 12, pp. 31–44.

This article gives an indication of how difficult quality-of-life research can be.

Opit, L. 1991, 'The Measurement of Health Service Outcomes', in W.W. Holland, R. Detels, & G. Knox (eds), *Oxford Textbook of Public Health*, vol. 2, 2nd edn, Oxford University Press, Oxford, ch. 10.

Richardson, J., Hall, J., & Salkeld, G. 1996, 'The Measurement of Utility in Multiphase Health States', *International Journal for the Technological Assessment of Health Care*, vol. 12, pp. 151–62.

Walker, S.R. & Rosser, R.M. 1993, *Quality of Life Assessment: Key Issues in the 1990s*, Kluwer Academic, Dordrecht.

This book is recommended for its thoughtful consideration of the many complex issues involved in this area of research.

Weinstein, M.C., Read, J.L., MacKay, D.N., et al. 1986, 'Cost-Effectiveness Choice of Antimicrobial Therapy for Serious Infection', *Journal of General Internal Medicine*, vol. 1, pp. 351–63.

CHAPTER 7

Personal Interviews

In questionnaire surveys (discussed in chapter 3), an important principle is to limit the data collected to those defined in the protocol. Often research respondents only need to tick the appropriate box in a questionnaire sent to them through the mail. The same questionnaire can also be 'administered' by a research assistant who asks the questions and ticks the boxes. This is probably the form taken by most personal interviews in the public health literature. But personal interviews cover a range of designs from 'tick-the-box' questionnaires to in-depth interviews, in which the people being interviewed have considerable control over what is recorded in the interview. What these various designs have in common is that people are asked by another person for their views. In this chapter we contrast two forms of personal interview: the structured personal interview and the in-depth personal interview.

The structured personal interview

Questionnaire surveys are relatively cheap and incorporate well-tested methods for ensuring that the data collected are not biased by the opinions of the interviewer. Collecting this data through a personal interview puts both of these advantages at risk. Unfortunately, the reasons for researchers choosing to do a personal interview are seldom reported. Sometimes they are obvious. Personal interviews can be used to extend a survey sample, as in the study of Kirkman-Liff and Mondragon (1991), who supplemented a telephone survey study of Hispanic Americans with personal interviews conducted, where necessary, in Spanish. This ensured representation of poor Spanish-speaking Hispanic people who were less likely to have telephones. The health status of this group was lower than that of other respondents.

A personal interview may also be necessary for taking physical measurements. Rissel and Russell (1993) supplemented a telephone interview on heart disease risk factors in a Vietnamese community in Sydney with a personal interview to measure blood pressure and cholesterol levels. In the process, the response rate dropped from 79 per cent to 48 per cent. A response rate as low as this poses problems for generalisability.

In contrast, face-to-face interviewing can be used to improve response rates. Interviewers may knock on doors of selected homes, often over weekends, asking a selected member of the household to participate. Interviewers fill in the questionnaire and take it away with them. Some researchers make use of 'omnibus' surveys, buying space for a set of questions in a larger survey conducted by commercial market-research firms. An example of this is a study of smoking prevalence by Hill and White (1995). In the 55 per cent of cases where an interview could not be conducted because of refusal or absence, replacements were found in other households. Such designs deliver large samples: the Hill study had 6046 respondents. In large questionnaires about general health issues, respondents are usually unaware of the purpose of individual questions. Smokers from socially disadvantaged groups might have been less keen to participate in the Hill study had they known that one of the options under consideration was increased taxes on tobacco, a measure seen as particularly effective in changing the smoking behaviour of lower income earners.

Despite personal approaches, response rates can remain low. This does not mean that the study is worthless, as researchers may be doing the best they can under difficult circumstances. An example is a British study of the relationship between gender, class, and smoking behaviour by Graham (1994). The researchers approached 1382 mothers living in Nottingham and Coventry; 66 per cent agreed to participate. Graham argues that the inclusion of questions on smoking behaviour as one part of a survey of the experiences of mothers with young children is likely to have encouraged accurate reporting of smoking behaviour but it may also have contributed to a response rate that might otherwise have been even lower.

This raises the problem that public health studies often involve the disclosure of information on what might be termed 'irresponsible' health behaviour — for example, overuse of alcohol or drugs. What is at issue is people's failure to 'comply' with good advice. Few of us are keen to display our own backsliding, and this may result in failure to 'comply' with the study as well. Researchers reporting on an abortive effort to study adolescent patients' non-compliance with treatment for diabetes note that medical non-compliance is 'a fertile and interesting topic for empirical research, if only we could get subjects to comply' (Roberts & Wurtele 1980: 171).

In the structured personal interview, issues of method remain identical to those discussed under questionnaire surveys, except that respondents persistently talk to the interviewer. In a case-control study of the exposure to environmental toxins of mothers of children born with congenital limb abnormalities (Kricker et al. 1986), it was impossible to prevent mothers from discussing their children, and interviewers could not be blinded to the case-control status of cases. Such breakdown of study protocol raises the problem of interviewer bias, which is defined in John Last's *A Dictionary of Epidemiology* (1995) as 'systematic error due to interviewers' subconscious or conscious gathering of selective data'.

In some studies, rigid limiting of interaction between interviewer and respondent may result in frustration for the reader when an extensive study seems to yield rather obvious (albeit reliable) results. Blaze-Temple and others (1988) demonstrated that parental non-compliance with measles vaccination for young children was associated with lower family income and parental apathy and fear. We are left wondering whether parents might have had something more useful to say about this problem had they been given more latitude than the ninety-six items in the structured questionnaire allowed.

Interestingly, interviewers conducting rigidly structured surveys sometimes come out of the interview saying that an off-the-cuff comment made by the person being interviewed was more valuable than the ticked boxes on the questionnaire form. Jylhä (1994) tape-recorded structured interviews on self-rated health and showed that respondents seldom opted for one or another of the set alternatives but preferred to describe and explain their views. One 85-year-old woman, when asked about her health state, described herself as more or less healthy except for a leg prosthesis, which caused difficulties without making 'much trouble'. While not completely healthy, she had never been really ill and had outlived most of her age peers. She was better able to explain how she saw her health than she was able simply to categorise it. Such answers can cause methodological complications for analysis but may be highly relevant to the problem. How might researchers respond? Wilson and co-workers (1993) included open-ended questions in a survey of Greek-Australians' health attitudes. Presumably because of the problem of interviewer bias in recording (or inventing?) data, they added a cryptic note: 'A proportion of each interviewer's allocated subjects were separately contacted by telephone to verify the interview' (p. 216). In a study of knowledge of cardiovascular risk by Frank and others (1993), study participants were asked open-ended questions like, 'In your opinion, is there anything a person can do to keep from having a heart attack or stroke?' Researchers merely coded responses according to preset categories.

Siegel and others (1989) went further. Interviewers talked participants through a series of questions on resistance to sexual assault, a delicate issue for which the response rate (68 per cent) was perhaps higher than might be expected. The study was conducted in Los Angeles with one catchment area being predominantly Hispanic American. Bilingual interviewers used filter questions to identify people who had experienced sexual assault and who had resisted. They were then simply asked, 'What did you do?'. Verbatim comments were recorded, and content analysis was conducted independently by three raters. Differences in interpretation were resolved through consensus. The six resistance strategies — talking, reasoning, denying any sexual interest, loud or angry talking, fleeing, and physical fighting — reduced the probability of assault, but the use of force by the assailant was more important in determining the outcome of an assault.

Verbatim comments can also deliver unexpected information. In 25 000 responses to a telephone survey of attitudes to lifestyle and health, including sexual behaviour, Nisbet and McQueen (1993) recorded 7000 verbatim comments. When analysed, those relating to AIDS showed victim-blaming attitudes, with extreme cases expressing punitive attitudes to high-risk groups. When it was realised that some interviewers were recording these comments more frequently than others, the protocol was changed to include a specific request for comments. The verbatim material was considered to be sufficiently important for separate publication.

Public health studies using structured personal interviews commonly focus on people's attitudes to, or knowledge about, the risk to health posed by certain personal behaviour (drug-use, diet) or environmental

> **Advantages of structured personal interviews**
> - Response rates may increase.
> - Unanticipated response may give valuable additional information.
>
> **Disadvantages of structured personal interviews**
> - They are more expensive.
> - Interviewer bias may be a problem.
> - Verbatim responses are more difficult to analyse.

effects. The aim is more often to define the factors that predict behaviour rather than to try to understand why people behave in the way they do. Typically the results feed into promotional campaigns, as did, for example, a large survey of health promotion priorities in communities in Sydney and Melbourne conducted by a commercial survey company (Pierce et al. 1985). It recommended increased promotional activity focused on cholesterol, exercise, and weight, similar to the mass-media campaigns directed at smoking and drink-driving.

In studies of this kind, the interviewer ideally becomes an instrument for filling in a questionnaire. This is the direct opposite of what happens with the in-depth interview.

The in-depth personal interview

Many researchers who have conducted in-depth interviews have had the experience of hearing a voice on the radio, or seeing a photograph in the press or a familiar face on the street, and immediately recognising the person with warmth and affection, only then remembering that they met the person when conducting a research interview. This cord of attachment between researcher and respondent resembles that between clinician and patient and is the special mark of in-depth personal interviews. As we shall see, these researchers see the issue of interviewer bias in a very different way, but let us first turn to some examples of such studies before outlining the methodological principles.

If we are interested in the reasons why women do not present for cancer-screening, a problem that has been with us for a long time, we may have found an Australian study by Irwig and others (1991) in the literature, which focused on women's perceptions of screening mammography. Their structured telephone survey was presented as a study of women's health. From their results, they argued that promotional messages to encourage screening should aim to correct misconceptions about cancer-screening — for example, by making older women more aware of their vulnerability to breast cancer. They did not attempt to show, in detail, why this problem arises.

A subsequent study done in the USA (Gregg & Curry 1994) provides a contrast. This in-depth interview study conducted in Atlanta, Georgia, focused on women who are 'underserved' by screening activities for breast and cervical cancer. The assumption of this study was that the problem lies in patients and clinicians having two distinct cultures. Middle-class, educated doctors, many of whom are White, see screening in biomedical terms. Women visiting the clinics are generally African-American, of lower socio-economic status, and with little education. The biomedical view is more familiar to us, but we have little idea of how these women perceive cancer-screening. From the anthropology literature, the researchers took the notion of the explanatory model — that is, a model that explains the way in which a person interprets disease and makes sense of a condition. From neighbourhood clinics, they enrolled eighty-nine African-American women over the age of forty years. While the interviews had a structured component (most interviews collect at least demographic data in this way), the major aim was to allow the women to express, in their own words, the way in which cancer and the threat of cancer impacted on their lives. The interviews lasted between 30 and 60 minutes and were tape-recorded where women agreed to this.

The women's explanatory model saw cancer-screening as a way of identifying the disease that would inevitably kill them; they saw little in the way of cure. The diagnosis caused distress that might kill a woman even faster, and treatment could increase poverty and erode health even further. In the light of this understanding, the question is not why some women do not get screened but why any get screened at all. Their recommendation was that prevention programs should promote contact with women who have survived cancer, but they noted that the advice from these women might well contradict medical advice. They recommended further study of African-American women from higher socio-economic groups and women from other ethnic groups.

In this case, the professional view was taken for granted, but it could also have been the subject of further interviews. In a study of chronic fatigue syndrome by Woodward and others (1995), researchers interviewed not only people with the syndrome but also the doctors treating them. Teasing out and explaining divergent opinions are often features of in-depth interviews. Pitts and others (1995) studied reactions to repeated sexually transmissible disease (STD) infections in Zimbabwe. Thirty men and thirty women attending a clinic for further treatment of new infections after having had at least one previous infection were randomly selected from clinic attenders. The study provided a simple tabulation of differences in the views of men and women. Men were not changing sexual behaviour to prevent infection, and women felt powerless to change this behaviour. The researchers identified the cause of the problem as cultural norms governing sexual behaviour and the stigma of infection.

Differences between the perceptions of men and women are also evident in a study by Becker and Nachtigall (1994), which records responses to the risk of infertility treatment. Participants, who had undergone or were undergoing fertility treatment, included 132 couples and eleven women interviewed without their partners. Topics discussed included the process that led to infertility treatment, experience of the treatment itself, as well as related events, feelings, and experiences. Cultural assumptions about parenthood (being 'born to be a mother') had a strong influence on perceptions of risk from the treatment. Although women were more aware than men of the risk involved, they were more prepared to take that risk.

Brown's study (1992) of interpretations of the childhood leukemia cluster in Woburn, Massachusetts, is a good example of a study that draws data from a range of sources. At issue was the relationship of the incidence of childhood leukemia to toxic waste leaking into the water supply. A civil suit had been taken against the company held responsible for the leaks. Data included two sets of interviews with litigants, and interviews with community activists, litigants' lawyers, public health officials, environmental officials, and public health researchers. In addition, data were drawn from legal documents and public meetings, and analysed in the light of evidence from archival sources and research from similar sites. All material was coded for themes from the existing literature and for themes emerging from the material collected. As a result, Brown could document a process of negotiation, through which the community role gradually became accepted by the public health agencies. The conflict, Brown argues, derived from a divergence between popular (lay) epidemiology and the views of scientific experts. Brown notes the irony that popular epidemiology closely resembles the methods used in the nineteenth century by John Snow, the founder of 'shoe leather' epidemiology, to close off the Broad Street pump and prevent the spread of cholera.

Let us end with a study that gives extensive information about the way in which researchers analyse data. The study by M.H. Kearney and co-workers (1994) focused on women in California who were addicted users of crack cocaine. Since these women were seen as less than ideal mothers, their children were often removed from their care by expensive legal procedures, with the additional public expense of then providing foster care. The literature review discussed various studies of heroin-users as mothers, but these focused on psychopathology or abnormal family interactions. Results of other studies were conflicting. There were no reports on how women in these circumstances actually go about caring for their children. Their own study started with a series of questions:

1 What are crack users' goals and standards for mothering?
2 What strategies do women who smoke crack use to care for children?
3 How does mothering vary under different conditions and at different levels of involvement in drugs?

The women interviewed were contacted through key informants from previous studies, using chain referrals. After screening over the telephone, sixty-eight mothers were interviewed for 1–3 hours in a place of their choice. They were invited to 'tell their stories' as they wished. The women, rather than the researchers, were seen as the 'experts' on the topic, and it was accepted that the researchers could not be seen as having a disengaged point of view. The research task was to examine 'shifts and trajectories of experience, the influences that affect identities, and participants' perceptions of events that change the course of processes such as mothering and drug use' (Kearney et al. 1994: 353). Differences in women's accounts were accepted as being expressions of their individuality and different social circumstances.

Mothering and drug-use were found to be incompatible activities, but mothers employed a range of strategies to separate them. They were intensely proud of their children, whom they defended from the drug life and its effects. The mothering outcome was influenced by an interactive complex of social and economic conditions. A woman is quoted as saying:

> It's a cycle. It's a cycle and it's vicious. And it beats us down. It's a system that takes poor people that have grown up poor and have no education and no skill like myself and it's like you don't believe there's ever a way out. So you turn to drugs because there's so much fucking pain. Then you lose these beautiful children. You have more pain. You use more drugs. You may try, but the court system eventually will beat you down. It's the same system that beat your mother down is gonna beat you down.

In a study of this kind, it is clearly more appropriate to talk about study 'participants' than to use the term 'respondents', which is common in studies using structured personal interviews.

Some practical principles

There is a series of steps that describe the methods commonly used in in-depth interview studies.

Let us now turn to a more detailed explanation of the various steps involved. Since the first two steps form the basis of a successful in-depth study, they are discussed in more detail.

Defining the research problem

A common theme in in-depth interview studies is that researchers have a research problem but do not know what is causing the problem. Researchers are also usually less concerned about controlling people's behaviour and more concerned with understanding why they do what they do. So, for example, there are various possible explanations for 'non-compliance' with medical advice. It may be that patients are too anxious to hear what their doctors say, or doctors may lack communication skills. Alternatively, patients may choose to ignore what they hear; they may simply be acting irrationally (from a medical perspective); or they may have their own good reasons for

> **Steps for in-depth interviewing**
> 1 Define a significant research problem.
>   • Conduct a literature review.
> 2 Select participants:
>   • for diversity or
>   • to represent groups likely to be most affected.
> 3 Collect data.
>   • Interview participants.
>   • Transcribe material.
> 4 Analyse data.
>   • Define categories for analysis and code data.
>   • Develop a preliminary explanation that makes sense of data collected, including deviant cases.
> 5 Select additional participants, diversifying the sample to take account of issues emerging from analysis or from interviews.
>   • Collect data to saturation for each new category.
> 6 Write an account that explains what is happening.

their actions. Drawing on common sense, we need to go to patients and ask them to tell us about it.

Researchers taking this common-sense approach need to distinguish carefully between personal chats and interview research. What then are the distinguishing marks of in-depth personal interviews? The first requirement is that the research should have the potential to contribute to public health by adding to our knowledge or testing knowledge about which we are unsure. Since few public health problems are new, we need to conduct a literature review to see what is already known. The synthesis of existing knowledge from meta-analyses (see chapter 10) is useful here. A systematic review of the literature is probably necessary for all research, but here it serves the additional purpose, as we shall see below, of contributing to the generalisability of results.

Defining a research problem, or a set of questions (as in the study of mothers using crack cocaine), is the in-depth study's equivalent of stating a hypothesis. Researchers may not know enough to be able to limit data-collection to specific variables. Instead they want to know what is going on. This does not mean that in-depth interviews are preliminary studies, useful only for generating hypotheses for later quantitative studies. In fact, most research occurs in cycles. We may start with an epidemiological survey that answers some questions but raises others. The next step may then be to conduct an in-depth interview study that provides further information. In turn, this may lead to a randomised control trial or another in-depth study, and so on.

Selecting study participants

With a research problem defined, the next step is to identify the groups of people most relevant to the topic and persuade them to join the study. Researchers are less interested in distribution across a population and more concerned with a detailed understanding of people's experience. Sometimes it is obvious where to start. Boutté (1990) was interested in the way in which people who have a parent with Machado-Joseph disease live with the 50-per-cent chance of inheriting this rare disease. She enrolled participants at three annual clinics of the International Joseph Disease Foundation in California. Similarly, if we are interested in health aspects of tattooing, we start with people who have tattoos. Houghton and others (1995) enrolled 130 people from a local tattoo studio and a further seventy-two from advertisements in community newspapers and on local radio.

If a problem is more widespread, it makes good sense to focus on groups in which we know the problem to be most evident. Wyn (1994) saw young women as a significant group for the study of sexually transmissible disease: they are beginning to be sexually active, and unsafe sex carries the risk of, among other problems, infertility. They interviewed ninety-five young women in Melbourne from a stratified sample of groups with relevance to health services provision (rural, outer-urban, inner-urban, homeless, Koori). A Koori (indigenous) research assistant helped negotiate recruitment from Koori communities; other young women were recruited through youth services, organisations, and schools.

The Wyn study relied on volunteer participation. Lupton and others (1995) also recruited volunteers and then selected people for interview. The study focused on the problem that Australia has a high rate of HIV antibody testing but a disproportionate number of these tests are conducted on 'low-risk' groups. A self-selected sample overcame the difficulties, practical and ethical, of identifying patients referred for the test. Given the emotional context of HIV testing, they preferred to interview people who had had a chance to reflect on the experience and who were willing to volunteer information. A poster displayed in a range of settings in Sydney attracted a diversity of respondents, resulting in 180 telephone calls. They also identified some participants through snowballing techniques, in which respondents are asked to contribute the names of other possible participants. They then selected for interview forty-one people from 'low-risk' groups, a sample stratified by gender, age, and reasons for having the test. The most common reason given for the test was that the person 'just wanted to know', but underlying this response were the symbolic uses of the test, such as demonstrating responsible behaviour towards a new sexual partner.

Selecting a heterogeneous sample is appropriate if what is in question is the consistency of views across a general population. Dicker and Armstrong's 1995 study of patients' views of priority-setting in health care took, as its starting point, the argument (much used by economists and health administrators) that the distribution of health-care resources should reflect the priorities of local communities. They selected participants to represent the mix of ethnic and social class characteristics of a London general-practice setting. Patients invited to participate in the study were given a list of nine services and asked to return two or three days later to discuss their own priorities. The sixteen participants found it difficult to assign priorities, being reluctant to express views based on self-interest. They were not persuaded of the need to ration health care at all, with one participant commenting: 'Well for starters there shouldn't have to be these decisions to be made!'. The authors point out that these people might have been persuaded to tick a preference box in a survey, but it would have reflected more what they perceive the needs of others to be rather than their own preferences. This underlines the value of one-to-one interviews, and the problem with questionnaires, when we cannot assume that researchers and participants interpret an issue in the same way.

There is a clear contrast between these studies and structured surveys. Study participants are selected to fit certain categories, and study populations can be small by comparison. It is often difficult to see from research reports how researchers decided on what was to count as an adequate 'sample'. Indeed, many researchers using these methods argue that they cannot specify how many people they need to interview before the study commences. If so, how do they know when to stop? Part of the answer lies in the arguments of Glaser and Strauss (1967) on 'saturation' of a sample, but the decision on sample size is intimately connected with the way in which data are collected and analysed.

Collecting data

When conducting in-depth interviews, it would be very unusual for researchers to disguise the topic in which they are interested. More commonly, the interviewer will outline the problem and then ask participants to talk about their own experiences or views. Some structured questions may be asked, but interviewers usually choose when to ask questions, in language adjusted to suit the participant. Interviews may take several hours. The data collected may include tape-recorded interviews, notes by interviewers, or other relevant material. In general, interview data are transcribed and filed together with relevant notes and background material.

An important difference with structured surveys should be noted here. The researcher is intimately involved in the process of collecting data and later in interpreting the material. Indeed, without a structured set of interview questions, the researcher *is* the research instrument. This makes data-collection a skilled task, and it is common for interviews to be conducted by the researchers themselves rather than by research assistants.

Analysing data

Analysis starts as the first data are collected, with researchers sorting data for their relevance to the research problem. Initial categories for sorting may be those identified in the literature review, but other categories emerge from participants' accounts. Methods for sorting data are intended to make it easier to retrieve data under particular categories from the mass of material that accumulates. The simplest method may be to cut up the transcript and file the material under separate headings, but this may prove to be cumbersome if the same lines of text have to be filed in more than one category. Researchers can also attach codes to the text itself, with methods for doing this ranging from underlining of text in different colours to using computer programs that store codes for specified lines of text.

The coded material is used to develop an explanation of the nature of the problem or the *quality* of an experience — hence the term 'qualitative data-analysis'. These accounts are usually written in everyday language with verbatim quotes giving insights into the views held by participants. Any data that do not fit the explanation ('deviant cases'), have to be identified and the difference explained. When researchers have sufficient material to be able to explain what is going on, and when new data are not contributing to any further understanding, the category is 'saturated' and data-collection ceases.

Selecting additional participants

If early analysis shows that there are important differences between groups of people in the study that cannot be explained, further data have to be collected from additional participants to explain the differences. When participants offer new insights during interviews, new categories for analysis are added, and different participants may need to be interviewed to the point of data saturation for each new category.

While this to-and-fro collection of data is a time-consuming task, the bulk of material that accumulates from each interview is large, leading to rapid saturation of categories. Small sample sizes are therefore common. It is important to note here that it is not sample size *per se* but the convincing nature of the account of that data that determines the methodological rigour of the study.

Writing the account

The aim of data-analysis is to develop an account that persuades the reader that rigorous methods have been used for gathering and analysing the material, and that the researchers understand the problem. This task of demonstrating understanding is not one that can be accomplished in a few short paragraphs; the generalisability of the study requires further argument. Commonly this is done by locating the study within the context of the literature review. If the results of the study are in agreement with other studies conducted in different settings, and the agreement can be explained, the generalisability of the study increases. Alternatively, if there are significant differences, then these have to be explained so that it is clear to which settings the result *does* apply.

The task of analysis through explanation and argument often results in journal articles that are 5000–6000 words in length, far too long for medical journals. Editing the argument down to 2000 words is possible, but the risk is that the analysis will appear superficial and the conclusions impressionistic. One way of addressing this problem is to reduce the data to numbers by defining a system for grading categories. For example, McDonald and others (1996) developed explicit criteria for grading aspects of consultations in which patients were 'reassured' by a negative test result. Inter-observer variability in the grading process was measured, and differences were resolved by consensus. Data sets could then be represented in tabular form. It could be argued that such procedures are more rigorous, but they have also been described as being useful mainly for 'covering one's back' rather than for contributing anything new to the analysis (Daly & McDonald 1992).

Advantages and disadvantages

In-depth personal interviews deliver a very attractive product. While the cost per interview is high, overall sample sizes are smaller. A major problem is that the actual methods used for conducting this research are highly dependent on the research context. This means that it is difficult to write a how-to textbook about qualitative research methods. It also means that this method is as difficult to learn as any of the other methods described in this book. This is an important consideration for those researchers who think that the method of 'talking to people' is so close to what we do in everyday life that anyone can do it.

Issues of ethics

Before invading people's personal space, we might well ask ourselves whether it is necessary to do so. There may well be other methods that minimise intrusion, and especially in delicate situations, unobtrusive methods might be preferable (Kellehear 1993a & b). Where there are existing data that have not been fully analysed, surely it is better to ask whether the answer can be obtained from further analysis of these data (see chapter 9). This issue is particularly relevant to over-researched communities. People with HIV infection or with AIDS are one such group. Indigenous people are another.

If we feel that we can justifiably intrude into people's lives, we must consider the way in which we go about doing so. When conducting

> **Advantages of in-depth interviews**
> - A large amount of rich data is produced from each interview.
> - They enable a detailed understanding of why people do, or believe, what they do.
> - Differences between groups are explained.
> - They make easy reading.
>
> **Disadvantages of in-depth interviews**
> - They are expensive (if we consider the cost per interview).
> - The validity of the study is highly dependent on the skills of the interviewer or researcher.
> - There is no defined way of testing for bias, validity, and generalisability.
> - It is difficult to have the results published in medical journals.

structured personal interviews, it may appear as if issues of ethics related to interaction with participants is at least minimised. This perception may, in itself, pose a problem if researchers do not recognise that interviewers need training in dealing with research respondents in a sensitive manner, especially in the case of potentially distressing topics. Qualitative in-depth researchers conducting their own interviews may have a distinct advantage here over untrained research assistants focused on obtaining a high response rate. However, careful training in ethical principles is necessary at all stages of the research task, and not just during data-collection.

The practice of disguising the research problem is a troublesome issue. When researchers disguise the purpose of their study (describing a study as being about health in general rather than risky behaviour, for example) this may deliver a bigger sample. But is deception involved? Participants may be contributing to a study that will demonstrate ways of 'persuading' them to change their behaviour. Would they participate if they knew the purpose of the study? And, if not, is it ethical to withhold this information? In in-depth interviewing such disguise is largely impractical: researchers need to tell participants exactly what the study is about to allow them to respond freely.

This brings us to the point that communities have a major stake in the way in which they are represented in research findings. There is now a long-overdue recognition that community groups, previously preyed upon by unscrupulous or thoughtless researchers, need to have a say both in setting research priorities and in the conduct of research. Such considerations are enshrined in ethical guidelines such as the Australian National Health and Medical Research Council's guidelines for research on Aboriginal and Torres Strait Islander health (NHMRC 1991). In addition, researchers need to give careful thought to the benefits that individual participants and the community itself can expect to gain from both the research process and the study findings (Anderson 1996). Even where there is no one definable community, the time-consuming task of negotiating research with study participants and reporting the findings back to those study participants is a necessary one, albeit not one for which researchers gain any special credit from public health funding bodies (Wyn et al. 1996).

Recommended reading

Britten, N. 1995, 'Qualitative Interviews in Medical Research', *British Medical Journal*, vol. 311, 22 July, pp. 251–3.
An excellent, brief beginner's guide.
Glaser, B. & Strauss, A. 1967, *The Discovery of Grounded Theory*, Aldine, Chicago.
A classic text.
Lofland, J. & Lofland, L.H. 1984, *Analysing Social Settings: A Guide to Qualitative Observation and Analysis*, Wadsworth Publishing Company, Belmont, Calif.
A well-tried sociological text.
Mays, N. & Pope, C. 1995, 'Rigour and Qualitative Research', *British Medical Journal*, vol. 311, 8 July, pp. 109–12.
This is part of a set of overview articles published over successive weeks.
Miles, M. & Huberman, A.M. 1984, *Qualitative Data Analysis: A Sourcebook of New Methods*, Sage, Beverley Hills, Calif.
This outlines practical qualitative method, as seen by an evaluator.
Minichiello, V., Aroni, R., Timewell, E., & Alexander, L. 1995, *In-Depth Interviewing: Principles, Techniques and Analysis*, Longman Cheshire, Melbourne.
A clear introductory text covering all stages of the research process.
Morse, J.M. (ed.) 1992, *Qualitative Health Research*, Sage, Newbury Park, Calif.
An edited collection of classic studies.

National Health and Medical Research Council 1991, *Guidelines on Ethical Matters in Aboriginal and Torres Strait Islander Health Research*, AGPS, Canberra.

A good starting point for research in communities of any kind.

Silverman, D. 1985, *Qualitative Methodology and Sociology: Describing the Social World*, Gower, Aldershot, UK.

Strauss, A. & Corbin, J. 1990, *Basics of Qualitative Research: Grounded Theory Procedures and Techniques*, Sage, Newbury Park, Calif.

An updated classic sociological text.

CHAPTER 8

Focus Group Interviews

If personal interviews are useful in studying public health problems, but time-consuming, then why not interview people in a group? After all, the time spent on a single interview could be used to gain information from five, seven, or twelve participants. Perhaps we could even 'process' twenty participants at a time. This is a seductive idea. An enthusiastic advocate might also point out that some market-research companies routinely use group interviews, and their sales would indicate soon enough if this method were not worthwhile. The answer to such alluringly simple ideas is often 'Ah, yes, but . . . '. So too in this case.

Let us draw on what we know about conversations with groups of people. It is difficult with any group to confine discussion to one topic, and there will always be some people in the group who will dominate the discussion. Think about the last dinner party you attended or discussions during family meals. On the other hand, committees are a good example of controlled group discussions with a specific purpose. Committee structures have developed over centuries along with well-understood procedures for focusing discussion on the task. A committee meeting usually has an agenda and a chairperson who ensures turn-taking in the discussion, with decisions being reached through consensus. The members of a committee are there to represent particular points of view or interests, but membership can be based on divergent or similar views. A committee assessing research grants, for example, may emphasise divergence, with members representing a range of research perspectives as well as the institutions involved — from government and universities to community groups. Alternatively, members may be selected to represent the same perspective — for example, when a group of qualitative researchers meet to draw up a set of guidelines for the ethical conduct of qualitative research.

Conducting a focus group has a degree of overlap with committee procedures. A facilitator or moderator takes the role of chairperson, and a set of research questions takes the place of the agenda. The discussion of the group is *focused* on these questions — hence the name. Depending on the question to be answered, members are selected to represent divergent or similar interests. Unlike committees, the discussion is likely to be tape-recorded, with the researchers then analysing what happened during the discussion and drawing conclusions about what they have learnt. Of particular interest in focus groups is the way in which the different members of the group interact with each other and what this tells the researchers about the views that they hold.

Researchers working in marketing and advertising have used focus groups since the 1920s, and continue to do so (Templeton 1987). A sociologist, Robert Merton, used group discussion in the 1950s to analyse people's responses to wartime propaganda. Gradually this technique has found a place in a range of health research settings. In the 1980s it was fashionable to conduct consensus conferences to guide decision-making about 'runaway' medical technologies. In 1984, for example, the National Institutes of Health in the USA convened an expert panel to develop a consensus position on the use of diagnostic ultrasound in pregnancy. They heard testimony from other professionals and from the public, and recommended against routine screening. Consensus methods such as the 'Delphi process' and the 'expert panel' involve structured processes in which expert judgment is synthesised and then fed back to participants until consensus is reached (Jones & Hunter 1995).

This chapter is most concerned with the use of focus groups to *analyse* a public health problem, rather than simply reaching consensus about it. As with personal interviews, focus groups can be structured or relatively unstructured, but the focus group equivalent of an unstructured in-depth personal interview would lead to chaos. (Even the most open-ended of focus groups has to set limits on what is seen as relevant to the problem in order to have a coherent discussion.) Focus group studies can be preliminary, hypothesis-generating studies or studies in their own right that are conducted as a result of questions raised in earlier studies. Focus groups may be the only research method used, or they may be one of a range of methods used in one study.

The popularity of focus groups in public health research has been rising steadily. Some researchers see focus groups as a cheaper way of getting a large sample than the one-to-one personal interview. To educators used to working with a classroom full of children, focus groups are an obvious way of obtaining information about health attitudes that, in turn, will be useful in educating these children (Basch 1987). Fortunately, because focus groups are still a relatively unusual public health research method, researchers often explain why they chose to use this method. In contrast with the other methods discussed in earlier chapters, there is not a good supply of published studies that demonstrate what the method achieves across a range of settings. Until anticipated benefit can be matched by proven achievement, a degree of caution is necessary.

Let us now turn to some examples to demonstrate how focus groups are used, starting with simple studies in which the focus groups are a supplement to quantitative studies, working up to more complicated studies in which focus groups are the only method used.

Some examples

The simplest use of focus groups is as a preliminary study to a survey, used for testing the relevance of study variables or the language used in a questionnaire. An example here is the study of sun-related attitudes and beliefs among Queensland schoolchildren (Lowe et al. 1993). Focus groups were used to identify the sun-protection factors that children saw as important, which were then included in the questionnaire. The aim of a study by Hall and others (1992) was to survey the public perception of the risks and benefits of alcohol. Focus groups and a pilot study were used for planning the 'study proper', which would be a face-to-face survey. The results of the focus groups were not reported.

The use of focus groups seems to provide a reasonable way of getting people to participate in studies that focus on the use of substances that are damaging to health; people may be much more at ease in 'confessing' to risky behaviour if they are in the company of other 'sinners'. The problem becomes a bit tricky if the substance is illegal. Let us look in detail at one study that used focus groups as part of a research strategy for studying illicit drug-use. Young illicit drug-users who are not at school or in treatment and who have not been arrested are often ignored in studies of drug-use. Random sampling techniques cannot be used as these young users are rare and difficult to locate.

Such arguments persuaded Spooner and Flaherty (1993) to conduct a study in Sydney starting with a ten-minute street intercept survey in which they asked 1000 young people about illicit drug-use. There are obvious methodological problems with a self-report study conducted under these circumstances, so they supplemented it with a telephone survey and focus group discussions. 'Respondents' for the focus groups were 'recruited' through advertisements (the use of this language is worth noting as it tends to indicate a more structured approach to research). Twelve focus group interviews were conducted with eighty-five young people, each paid A$30, at venues that were easily accessible and that had a relaxed atmosphere. The overall cost per respondent of the focus groups was calculated to be four times that of the street survey, but the groups did give respondents the opportunity to raise their own issues. One of the issues emerging from focus group discussion was the importance of parental example; the disapproving parent who smokes may lack credibility. When the moderator raised issues from the survey, the information obtained was more detailed. For example, while the survey showed that few of the young users had been arrested, the focus group showed that they did have experience with the police system, with the majority reporting that they had been harassed by police.

Group dynamics, a special feature of focus groups, meant that members challenged statements made by others in the group so that the reason for differences of opinion became clear. While the survey data showed differences between individual users, the focus groups showed light and heavy users to be consistently different in their responses. The researchers concluded that the focus groups were an important 'adjunct' to the quantitative surveys, but that the survey was a necessary part of substantiating and quantifying the 'impressions' formed in the group interviews.

Unlike illicit drug-use, cigarette-smoking is legal, but we tend to draw the line at children smoking. In many countries tobacco advertising directed at young people is unacceptable, but the question is whether tobacco advertising apparently directed at adults influences young people's smoking behaviour. Since focus groups are used in market research to assess responses to a product for advertising campaigns, it makes sense to use the same method to assess the impact of cigarette advertising on young people.

Hastings and colleagues (1994) conducted a study in Glasgow of a cigarette-advertising campaign featuring a cartoon character, Reg. Three separate surveys were conducted in addition to a focus group component, which involved eighteen group interviews with 117 people aged 10–55 years. The groups were structured to be homogeneous with respect to age, gender, smoking status, and socio-economic status. 'Respondents' were recruited by door-to-door canvassing and were paid for their attendance at a 'prearranged venue'. Discussions with children lasted about five hours, which gave time for the children to relax and for complex interviewing techniques to be used, including games in which the children matched products and slogans. All interviews were tape-recorded and transcribed.

In this study, three of the researchers were working in marketing and one in education. They note: 'With hindsight, the interviews were probably longer and more elaborate than necessary and the same data could have been retrieved in half the time' (p. 933). Although there is little evidence of in-depth analysis of the data, they showed that Reg caught the attention of young children rather than adults, with the appeal of the advertisement being related to an association of the brand with status or fashion. Thus the study achieved its purpose: the voluntary code governing tobacco advertising was being contravened and Reg was withdrawn. The headline to the *British Medical Journal* editorial on the study (Chapman 1994) attributes the success of stopping the advertisement to the qualitative component of the study.

Another study of the impact of tobacco advertising on young children (Aitken et al. 1985) used focus groups alone. Again the aim was to demonstrate that the voluntary code of practice on tobacco advertising was being broken. Two of the three authors came from advertising research and the third from psychology. They chose to use focus groups because they believed that children do not respond well to structured questionnaires and are more forthcoming with their comments in groups than in a one-to-one setting. According to complex attitude research, discussion is seen as important in exploring areas rather than obtaining specific but superficial answers. Minor modifications to the questions were also possible when interviewing children from very different socio-economic backgrounds.

The twenty-four focus groups with children only lasted 75 to 90 minutes and were coherent with respect to age, gender, and socio-economic locality (inner-city working-class and middle-class suburban). Children were asked to comment on a range of advertising material, including cigarette advertisements. Measures of agreement and disagreement were taken by show-of-hands voting, and analysis focused on consistency within sub-groups and across the sample as a whole. Area and gender division were found to be unimportant, and the consensus reached within age groups became the focus of analysis. The results showed a decrease in moral condemnation of smoking with age. There was evidence to suggest that advertising aimed at young adults was also attractive to young teenagers (14–16-year-olds).

Both of these studies addressed essentially the same problem, but they did so in different ways, each providing a clear description of the research process. Given the limited analysis of the data collected, we are left wondering whether perhaps a simpler design would have sufficed. In contrast, a simple, pragmatic study of illicit drug-use (Dodding & Gaughwin 1995) was conducted by researchers working in drug and alcohol studies in Western Australia and South Australia. At issue was the potential impact of needle- and syringe-vending machines. The focus groups were seen as a means of obtaining the views of users in a non-threatening environment. Injecting drug-users were recruited by circulating leaflets through exchange programs, drug-user organisations, and pharmacies. Only four focus groups were held with twenty-four drug-users, who were paid A$20 each. There was also one focus group with seven workers in the field. The two groups had largely similar responses.

While the study collected data from only a limited number of participants, it made good use of the material collected. Researchers analysed answers to pre-set questions and identified themes in the discussion, with particular attention being paid to themes that provoked agreement or discord. There was general agreement that drug-users would go to vending machines but that the machines should be carefully located after discussion with local groups to minimise risk to minors who are not using drugs. The researchers were cautious about their conclusions because of the small number of interviews and the self-selected nature of the people interviewed, but they argued that there was good reason to believe that injecting drug-users would make use of vending machines. These have since become a common feature in Australia.

A minimalist approach is also a feature of many studies done from a consumer perspective. Consumer health agencies spend a fair portion of each day discussing people's health problems, and research involving focus groups may require only small extensions to their everyday practice. Since much of this research appears only in reports for local distribution, it is gratifying to find a few examples making their way into the public health literature. A study of access to health care for children in low-income families by the Brotherhood of St Laurence in Melbourne (Taylor 1994) was based on two focus group discussions held in low-income areas. One was with mothers whose children attended a local kindergarten and the other with a new mothers' group, which met in a local health centre. The women were asked simply about difficulties in accessing health services for their children, and the most frequently cited problem was the cost of that care.

At their best, studies involving consumer groups can lead directly to change, as in a study of the hazards and risks for children living on farms (Wolfenden et al. 1992). This study used a check-list drawn up by a local action group on rural safety and tested it in focus groups with a local farming community. The researchers argue that the check-list was readily implemented in a safety campaign because it had local relevance; the research process contributed to community action. It is worth noting that both the community-based studies were conducted in local settings; neither paid the people who came to the interview.

Focus group studies have been found useful as a way of consulting formally with a community. The Somerset Health Authority in the United Kingdom set up eight panels of twelve local people each, representing a cross section of the community (Bowie et al. 1995). The panels discussed issues facing the health authority, with the group setting providing the opportunity for people to debate community needs. The panels had the potential to contribute to decision-making by the health authority. Brown (1995) conducted groups for a similar purpose in Hull. Eleven meetings were conducted, drawing on volunteers and pre-existing groups. Participants were asked, 'If you had £1 million to spend on health services, what would you spend it on?'. As in the interview study of Dicker and Armstrong (1995) discussed in the last chapter, further funding for the National Health Service was the preferred option rather than prioritisation of spending. Such agreements add weight to both studies. However, participants were prepared to identify fertility treatment as an area of lower priority: 'I think if something's got to go, test tube babies can'.

Some communities are much less accessible than these, and their views may be much more difficult to understand. Perhaps because, in order to gain this more detailed understanding, researchers need the active cooperation of the people they interview, it becomes more common for the people they interview to be referred to as 'participants'. An example is the study by Hamid and others (1995) of the beliefs and practices relating to pregnancy and the birth process of Malay, Chinese, and Indian squatter women living in the areas surrounding Kuala Lumpur City. A household survey was used to define the topics for focus group discussion and to identify ten women (including Malay, Indian, and Chinese women) to participate in the groups. What was at issue was a more detailed understanding of the culturally derived ways in which women cared for their health during this period.

As we move towards the more complex end of the spectrum of focus group studies, studies of the HIV/AIDS epidemic become more frequent. An early study (Chapman & Hodgson 1988) set the scene for much of this work in Australia. It focused on condom-use, with people recruited from a range of settings in which a casual sexual partner might be sought (hotel bars, discos, drop-in centres, and so on). The researchers describe their recruitment methods as based on common sense. Focus group leaders were given a list of topics to do with condom-use, which they raised if the topic did not come up spontaneously in discussion. The interviews showed that people clearly understood the risk of AIDS but that they believed that they could identify safe sexual partners from their appearance. Since they saw condoms as the equivalent of 'showers in raincoats', there was an urgent need to 'conceptually reposition the condom', as the researchers quaintly put it. As we now know, this has been a central concern of the AIDS-prevention strategy.

Researchers working in AIDS research have had little option but to confront the complexities of cultural beliefs and practices. Konde-Lule and colleagues (1993) used focus groups to study knowledge, attitudes, and practices with respect to AIDS in the Rakai district in Uganda. Community leaders were asked to invite participants to thirty-five focus groups. Categories for the groups included married men or women, manual workers, barmaids, youths, community leaders, police, business persons, and traditional healers. Again, the risk of transmission of HIV was well understood, but the preferred prevention measure was limiting sexual partners rather than condom-use. These findings are largely in agreement with the focus group study of factory workers in Kinshasa, Zaire, conducted by Irwin and others (1991), where the result of the research was a counselling and educational program for the workers.

The difficulties of conducting research about private topics in culturally diverse groups in a language not spoken by the researchers cannot be underestimated (for an outline of the difficulties of this kind of research, see Yelland & Gifford 1995). A study of sexual choice among 'high-risk' Black and Hispanic women (Kline et al. 1992) gives a fine description of a sensitively designed study. These researchers conducted sixteen focus groups with 134 women from drug-treatment centres and community agencies in New Jersey. Counsellors at the centres had identified women who were either intravenous drug-users or HIV positive, and when approached, 90 per cent agreed to participate. An outreach worker was used to recruit women who were sex partners of current intravenous drug-users.

Interviews, conducted by highly trained interviewers of the same gender and ethnic background, used a flexible protocol. They asked questions in their own words and timed questions to fit in with the flow of conversation. The sixteen interviews each lasted for two hours and produced 900 pages of transcript. All speakers were identified on the transcript. This is no easy task, as people in groups commonly speak over each other and voices can sound very similar on tape. The mass of data was coded into categories representing general content as well as the women's responses. Themes or patterns of response were identified by clustering categories. They found that women were often able to insist on the use of condoms by using various strategies. They could take advantage of a partner's state of sexual arousal: 'You can get him real horney [sic], and then when the time comes you tell him he gets nothing unless he uses one' (p. 453). They could exploit cultural factors, like a male sense of responsibility for protecting the family, to encourage condom-use. This paper contains an excellent discussion of the extent to which these findings can be generalised to other communities.

Some practical principles

The conduct of focus groups has considerable overlap with the in-depth personal interview. The focus of discussion needs to be a clearly defined research problem. Focus groups are not easy or cheap when compared with most other methods. Typically, focus groups work best when people are more comfortable discussing a topic in a group, especially when interaction between group members provides a way of clarifying their views.

From the literature review or from experience in the field, researchers usually have a fair idea of the factors that are likely to explain the way in which different groups of people respond to a problem. In the cigarette-advertising study, for example, inner-city working-class children were compared with middle-class suburban children These distinctions represent preliminary data categories, and they form the basis for selecting the groups for interview.

The next choice is to decide whether the focus groups is to be a stand-alone study, in which case the findings will be interpreted in the light of other studies in the area. Alternatively, the focus group study can serve as a preliminary study, to define issues or test the language for a questionnaire. A focus group study can also follow a survey to provide a more detailed understanding of unexpected results.

In simple, pragmatic, or preliminary studies, it may appropriate to choose focus group participants so that the full range of different views is present in the same group. The aim then is to reach consensus. The interview schedule can be fairly structured, and data-analysis can be as simple as counting votes. This is often the approach used by researchers from marketing or advertising. It also seems to be favoured by quantitative researchers using the focus group as a preliminary study, or even as a way of adding 'spice' and the odd quote to an otherwise dull survey.

The more challenging approach is to select focus groups so that there are participants of similar backgrounds in any one group but with differences between the groups. In the study by Kline and others (1992) of sexual choice, for example, the researchers held separate groups for Black and Hispanic women who were intravenous drug-users, HIV positive, and sexual partners of intravenous drug-users. The focus in each group was to identify and talk through both the similarities and the differences in the views of participants.

The task of the interviewer is clearly of crucial importance. This person has to keep the discussion on target, while using a mental check-list of problems to be introduced in an appropriate manner at an appropriate time, but only if the participants do not themselves volunteer the information. Kitzinger (1994) argues that the role of the interviewer is to encourage as much interaction as possible. Thus the participants become 'co-researchers', taking the discussion into areas not anticipated by the researchers. If there is sharing of common experiences, the mode of discussion may be complementary; if case differences are explored, it may be argumentative. Both are of value. As these 'co-researchers' spark off responses in each other, an inexperienced interviewer could lose control of the direction of discussion. Here is one such exchange described by Kitzinger:

> some participants acted out the 'look' of an 'AIDS carrier' (contorting their faces, squinting and shaking) and others took evident delight in swapping information about the vast quantities of saliva one would need to drink before running any risk of infection. (You'd need to swallow 'six gallons', 'eight gallons', 'ten gallons' or 'bathe in it while covered in open sores'.) (Kitzinger 1994: 108).

One could imagine that a person who was HIV positive would find these descriptions distressing. If this happens, it is the interviewer's task to steer the discussion in such a way that the distress is resolved.

As with the in-depth personal interview, analysis involves sorting data into 'boxes', one for each of the pre-set categories. Further categories for analysis emerge from the discussion. Ideally, researchers need to continue the collection of data until each of these categories is saturated — that is, until any new data collected fail to add anything new to the analysis (Glaser & Strauss 1967). Sometimes in the delicate areas that are the topic of many focus group studies, practical constraints mean

---

Steps for focus group interviews
1 Define the research problem.
2 Define categories for selecting focus group participants.
3 Set up focus groups for:
   • homogeneity within each group or
   • diversity within each group.
4 Interview groups.
5 Define additional categories for analysis.
6 Develop an explanation of similarities and differences within each group and between groups.
7 Write an account that explains how people see or experience a problem.

that saturation of data is impossible. In the Kline study, for example, the researchers were only able to bring together four focus groups of women who were the sexual partners of intravenous drug-users.

The reporting of a study using an in-depth approach takes the form of a logical argument, explaining what was done and the conclusions of the study. Since interaction between focus group participants is part of the reason for choosing this method, one would expect to see this conversation reported. As is the case with in-depth interviews, verbatim quotes from transcripts tend to make research reports extremely long and difficult to publish in medical journals.

Advantages and disadvantages

Focus group interviews may be seen as cheaper than in-depth personal interviews because they produce a larger 'sample' per unit of interview time. This may well be true of simple, pragmatic studies in which interaction between respondents is ignored. However, if our aim is to take account of interaction and allow free-wheeling discussion between participants, then running the group and interpreting the data may take so much time that the cost advantage is lost. On the other hand, we do gain access to people discussing their agreements and differences about a problem, providing we can keep a hold on the discussion.

The data obtained are commonly described as 'rich' — and so they are. Unfortunately they can also provide an 'embarrassment of riches', with enough data to overwhelm the unwitting researcher. This is where research skill comes in. Focus groups may look like a common-sense way of collecting data by talking to people — something that anybody can do with a topic, a tape recorder, and a few friends. The problem becomes apparent when the data have to be analysed. It is at this stage that researchers often begin to realise that there is no easy route to good research, whatever the approach. Social science students are taught qualitative research skills in undergraduate or postgraduate courses. These skills cannot be acquired in a weekend workshop; nor will a user-friendly computer program do the analysis for you. As is demonstrated by many of the more complex studies cited, it is a good idea to have a well-trained social scientist on the study.

As in the case of in-depth interviewing, issues of validity depend heavily on both the skill of the interviewer in conducting the interview and the skill of the researchers in synthesising the mass of data into a coherent account. Sometimes there will be uncertainty about the extent to which the experience of one group of participants represents the experience of other, different groups. The literature review comes in useful here. The issue of generalisability has to be addressed by carefully arguing through the extent to which the results could apply to other groups. This is a difficult task, which many of the studies outlined earlier simply evaded.

The advantages and disadvantages of focus group research are similar to those of in-depth interviewing, except that both advantages and disadvantages may be intensified by the additional complexity of the group interview.

Advantages of focus group interviews
- They produce a very much larger amount of rich data than one-to-one interviews.
- They can encourage people to speak about potentially embarrassing topics.
- People are allowed to debate differences or to express agreement.
- They are good at explaining differences and agreements between groups and within groups.

Disadvantages of focus group interviews
- There is a very high cost per interview.
- It is difficult to control a group while allowing free-wheeling discussion.
- It is difficult to identify different participants in transcription.
- Issues of validity and generalisability are complex.

Focusing on ethics

A bad dinner guest is one who raises contentious and potentially embarrassing issues for discussion at the dinner table. The other guests may get distressed or angry, and the evening could be ruined. But this is exactly what focus group interviewers do. How then are we to justify this behaviour as ethical research?

Perhaps if we pay our 'respondents', this distinguishes the relationship as different, but it raises the problem that people may feel obliged to 'perform' for the fee paid. Sometimes this payment is to cover travel costs to a venue that is convenient for the researchers rather than the study participants, and this may be unavoidable. Where, for example, could one interview a group of homeless people who do not use agency services? But payment may also be a way of getting reluctant participants to enrol in a study, and it is not clear what impact this has on the data they give us. An interesting variation on this theme is demonstrated by a study in which interviewers were 'given an incentive' (unspecified) for obtaining ten interviews with teenagers about drug-use (Levy & Pierce 1989). Many researchers conducting focus group studies start by establishing contacts in, and ties with, the community in which they are going to conduct their research. This takes time, but it resolves many of the problems of research ethics. It is more likely that interviews will be conducted in a setting that is convenient for the participants rather than the researchers and the issue of paying for travel is removed. If the research addresses an issue seen to be important to the community, people are more likely to want to participate in the study and a fee will be unnecessary. The research is more likely to benefit the community, rather than just the researchers.

Good relations between researchers and community groups can bring about changes in a research design that solve ethical problems as they emerge. Jeanne Daly (1997) described a study of women's perceptions of menopause in which groups were selected to represent key categories. In early discussions, women became distressed about intense differences in their views on hormone replacement therapy (HRT). The decision was taken to move to interviewing 'friendship groups'. One woman, who fitted a research category, was approached and asked to invite a number of like-minded friends — whom she thought would feel comfortable discussing a broad range of issues to do with menopause — to be interviewed in her home. This had the additional advantage that women who became distressed had a group of supportive friends at hand who would remain in contact after the interviewer went home. In a number of cases, the interviews led to the setting up of self-help groups to help other women in similar circumstances, thus directly benefiting both participants and community.

Having said this, we cannot overemphasise the problem of upsetting participants. There may well be a large number of people out there who want to talk about things that distress them, but there is nobody who will listen. Focus groups, like in-depth interviews, have the advantage that a good interviewer need say very little beyond defining the topic for discussion. In this way, the risk of compulsion or obligation is reduced: people tell what they want to tell. In fact, a hidden problem may be that some interviewers find it difficult to cope with the sad stories that they are told, and the interviewer may also need support (Kellehear 1989). Of the studies outlined in this chapter, the one that springs to mind is the study by Kline and others (1992), which contains page after page of quotes from women battling with the problems of drug-use or with being HIV positive. Here is one example, a comment from a woman who is HIV positive:

> I love him and I would feel bad that by not using a condom his infection would progress. A lot of people wonder how I can feel this way when he was the one who infected me. I don't know. He is the father of my son and I loved him (p. 451).

We owe a debt of gratitude both to the people who participated in this study and the interviewers who conducted it.

Recommended reading

Basch, C.E. 1987, 'Focus Group Interview: An Underutilized Research Technique for Improving Theory and Practice in Health Education', *Health Education Quarterly*, vol. 14, no. 4, pp. 411–48.

Glaser, B. & Strauss, A. 1967, *The Discovery of Grounded Theory*, Aldine, Chicago.
    A classic text on qualitative research.

Jones, J. & Hunter, D. 1995, 'Consensus Methods for Medical and Health Services Research', *British Medical Journal*, vol. 311, 5 August, pp. 376–80.
    This article discusses Delphi method.

Kitzinger, J. 1994, 'The Methodology of Focus Groups: The Importance of Interaction between Research Participants', *Sociology of Health and Illness*, vol. 16, no. 1, pp. 103–21.
    An excellent overview and critique.

Kitzinger, J. 1995, 'Introducing Focus Groups', *British Medical Journal*, vol. 311, 29 July, pp. 299–302.
    This is a brief, simple, good introduction.

Krueger, R. 1988, *Focus Groups: A Practical Guide for Applied Research*, Sage, London.
    A standard text written for decision-makers.

Merton, R. 1987, 'The Focused Interview and Focus Group: Continuities and Discontinuities', *Public Opinion Quarterly*, vol. 51, pp. 550–66.
Morgan, D. 1988, *Focus Groups as Qualitative Research*, Sage, London.
Another classic text.
Templeton, J.F. 1987, *Focus Groups: A Guide for Marketing and Advertising Professionals*, Probus, Chicago.
Thomas, S., Steven, I., Browning, C., et al. 1992, 'Focus Groups in Health Research: A Methodological Review', *Annual Review of Health Social Sciences*, vol. 2, pp. 7–20.

CHAPTER 9

Secondary Analysis

Until now, we have emphasised the *empirical* nature of public health research. But not all public health research is, has been, or needs to be empirical. One can analyse, or reanalyse, the data that others have collected. This is known as 'secondary analysis'. The range and quantity of potential data sources are truly remarkable. Data in the form of existing statistics may be retrieved from the data archives of local, state, or federal governments; from universities and hospitals; from businesses and other private organisations; or even from historical sources, such as old official records.

Too often social researchers feel that *original* research is about *going out* and surveying, interviewing, or observing people. But this is not necessarily the case. Originality is not simply about new data; rather it is about new insights. And fresh insights can be gained from almost any source, including other people's data. New relationships between the data, not noticed by the original researchers, may be discovered. New questions asked of old data may reveal new possibilities or may critically alter our understanding of the old conclusions.

Ever since written records were first kept, social researchers have been examining and re-examining them. Birth, deaths, and marriage records have been as useful to historians as they have been to public health researchers. But in public health research, concern with existing statistics has attracted the most attention, overshadowing the contributions of secondary analysts. However, as a methodology in general, secondary analysis is not confined to official records only. Newspapers, popular literature, letters, books, personal diaries — indeed almost anything found in a library or archive — can be the subject of this style of analysis. But secondary analysis of these sources involves more than simply reading these texts for their conclusions or insights; rather, it involves performing a content analysis of them.

Secondary analysis may serve two aims. On one hand, we can analyse the data source to recheck the original analysis, looking for strengths and weakness in the original operations and design of argument and evidence. For example, with statistical data, this may entail re-examining the methods of data-analysis. In narrative texts, such as social histories, letters, or newspapers, this may include a re-examination of the categories used in the original content-analysis. On the other hand, we can ask new questions of old data, leaving aside the original analysis and performing entirely new analysis on the data set. Once again, the data set may be numerical, as with existing statistics, but it may be in the form of a narrative text, such as with personal diaries, letters, or public documents. Let us look at these procedures more closely by reviewing some examples.

Some examples

The overwhelming majority of health studies based on secondary analysis tend to look for their data sources in very conventional areas. Allan Kellehear (1993a) found that the majority of sources used by these studies tended to be federal or state government sources of statistics alone. Particularly popular were figures from local departments of health, or their health insurance records of patient consultations and payments.

Key among the concerns of secondary-analysis researchers are infant and adult mortality figures. There are thousands of such studies, more than a few of which argue that such figures indicate the general health of the nation (Singh & Yu 1995). Some studies are fascinating for idiosyncratic reasons, such as the study by Walrath and others (1985), which looked at causes of death among female chemists. Others are of interest because of their topical nature — the study of firearm-related deaths by Alexander and others (1985), for example. However, many others debate perennial issues, such as the relationship between health and social class.

Typical of this tradition is Najman's (1993) study, which re-examines the relationship between health and poverty. In this study he employed age-standardised mortality rates, infant-mortality rates, and life-expectancy figures from government and academic sources. He argues that the disadvantages of using the idea of 'class' now outweigh the advantages, and suggests that we move to more precise indicators such as income or even membership of known disadvantaged groups, such as single mothers or the disabled.

Interesting variations on this common and dominating concern with class indices can be seen in the work of Hogg (1992), Hall (1986), and Bentham (1991). Hogg compared mortality rates for Australian Aborigines with indigenous peoples in the USA, Canada, and New Zealand, and found that the rates for Australia's indigenous people were uniquely worse. Neither existing information about risk and genetic factors nor psychosocial influences seem to explain this anomaly. In a novel twist on the use of mortality statistics, Hall examined the relationship of social class and survival on the S.S. *Titanic* by examining data from the Mersey Committee of Inquiry and from the White Star Line Company itself. Contrary to the findings of the inquiry, Hall found that class discrimination was the result of policy and some unsystematic exclusion by the crew, who favoured upper-class passengers in filling the life boats. Finally, Bentham examined perinatal mortality rates to assess the common belief that the Chernobyl fallout had effected these rates in England and Wales. He concluded that there was little evidence for this belief.

Meg Montague (1983) tackled a few ideas that are perhaps even more deserving of criticism. By re-examining figures from the Australian Bureau of Statistics, as well as those of departments of health and welfare, Montague challenged several ideas surrounding teenage pregnancy, dependency on government benefits, and unemployment during the period 1970–80 in Australia.

Focusing on another country and period, Tsey and Short (1995) examined figures from Ghana for the years 1898–1929 to investigate the health of expatriates, élites, and the poor during railway work in that country. Their data sources were from the Public Record Office (morbidity and mortality data), the Railways Annual Report (accident rates), annual reports of the Transport Department (for occasional descriptions of work environments and conditions), and some correspondence from senior officials and administrators of the day (for descriptions and records of conflict over occupational health and safety issues).

In the USA, Greenberg and Schneider (1994), in a fascinating challenge to a widely held popular and academic belief, demonstrate that young

Black males are no more the cause or likely victims of violence than any other age, gender or ethnic group. Examining the mortality rates of three marginal urban areas, they show that *all* groups in such areas have a higher risk of deaths from suicide, murder, drug-abuse, falls, fires, or poisoning. It may be that more Blacks live in such areas in the USA, but it is the areas themselves — that is, the physical and social risks engendered by such environments — and not the ethnicity, age or gender of particular people, that are the responsible factor.

A study from the USA, but about events in Japan, identifies a major source of death misclassification in Japanese mortality rates (Rockett & Smith 1993). The study's sources are from the Japanese Ministry of Health and Welfare, and from World Health Organisation mortality data, especially data classified under ICD-9 external cause rubrics (E-codes, which are the International Classification of Diseases codes for death from environmental causes). The rate of 'unintentional drownings' for Japanese women over forty-four years of age is excessive. Over the age of seventy-five, these rates exceed international comparisons by 7–15 times. Since intentional drowning is the third most common form of suicide among Japanese women, the rather extreme levels of 'unintentional' drowning for elderly women call for further scrutiny.

Medicare data have been used to examine dehydration morbidity among the American elderly (Warren et al. 1994); hospital in-patient data have been used to assess the issue of unnecessary surgery (Schacht & Pemberton 1985); the United States Fatal Accident Reporting System has been used to assess the relationship between car mass and fatality risk (Evans & Frick 1994); cancer registries have been used for innumerable research reasons, but Liff and others (1991) used them to determine whether increased detection has artificially inflated breast cancer incidence rates. Their answer, by the way, was partly 'yes' but mainly 'no'.

And apart from the lusty attractions of statistics, there have been many other studies employing non-numerical sources of data. Ashton (1988) re-examined the 'Health in Mersey' report; Blaze-Temple and others (1989) examined health legislation and its impact on addiction policy. Others have done similar work with legislation, but have looked for implications for AIDS and women (Neave 1989) or tobacco-use (Peachment 1984; Woodward et al. 1989).

Koutroulis (1990) looked at sexist ideas about women in undergraduate textbooks for medical students and discussed the implications of these embedded ideas for service-delivery to this patient population. Bammer and others (1995) employed ambulance service records to examine non-fatal heroin overdoses. And finally, Rainey and Runyan (1992) employed a content analysis of newspapers and compared this with medical-examiner records to assess completeness and accuracy of newspaper coverage.

Advantages and disadvantages

What drives all these researchers to analyse or re-analyse other people's data, or indeed, to employ data from unusual or non-numerical sources? Clearly this type of research has specific advantages. According to Kellehear (1993b: 53), there are basically four major advantages to secondary analysis work.

First, studying established record holdings, such as data held in archives or libraries, may provide a *comprehensive* data source. Secondary data can be collected through the retrieval of other researchers' data, as with census material or data sets lodged in data archives by other colleagues. As well as this secondary data, however, 'raw' data or primary data may also be collected, coded, and analysed for the first time. For example, good qualitative data can be collected by analysing personal documents such as letters or published interviews. Good quantitative data can be collected from annual reports of companies or hospitals, from newspapers, or merely by coding, typifying, and analysing narratives of illness that appear in popular literature. And along with primary and secondary sources of data, we can often find literature to support that data source in records existing alongside those data: the reports or articles that contain the original analysis, unpublished reports, or researchers' notes. If the data set is located in a university library, books and articles that support the research interest might also be found there. This is the closest one might get to 'one-stop shopping' in public health research.

The second advantage associated with secondary analysis is that often the data being analysed may be unique, either methodologically or historically. A study, for example, that has taken twenty years to complete, operating over four nations, and that has cost some several millions of dollars in funding constitutes work *and* data that are unique. This is not work that is easily repeated; the data set, therefore, is an important and perhaps ongoing source of secondary analysis. World Health Organisation data, or even one's local national census material, may fall into categories similar to this. Other data may have been collected a long time ago (centuries-old data, for example). They may focus on populations that no longer exist (the urban working class in nineteenth-century London, for example), or they may document unique environmental conditions (the bombing of Hiroshima, or conditions for nineteenth-century mine workers, for instance).

Third, existing records — whether they be from annual reports of the national Bureau of Statistics, from departments of social services or health, or from personal diaries — can supply good sources of longitudinal data. As long as the data have been documented and are extracted for analysis in a consistent way, these sources can supply information on individuals and populations spanning decades.

And finally, of course, as they are often permanent records, most of these sources are highly reliable — that is, they can be rechecked by others. Additionally, many of these data can be inexpensive to obtain and analyse. They may, in fact, be free, if obtained through the university library, for instance. Furthermore, if the data are purchased from a data archive, the cost can be nominal. Reliability and low cost make secondary analysis appealing to those interested in poorly funded research areas.

Advantages of secondary analysis
- It provides a potentially comprehensive source of data that is not necessarily confined to secondary sources alone.
- Data are often unique, either methodologically and/or historically.
- It often supplies good sources of longitudinal data.
- Data are highly reliable; that is, they are easily rechecked by others.
- It can be inexpensive.

However, not all key methodological concerns are addressed as easily as that of reliability. There are some important questions that go to the heart of the validity problem in secondary analysis. Roy Carr-Hill (1990), in a penetrating critical paper examining the measurement of inequities in health, summarises many of these concerns. Measures of social class — occupation, occupational prestige, income, education — are not necessarily comparable across time or internationally. Occupations attract different prestige, income, and educational requirements, depending on the period and local cultural influences.

This problem of valid categorisation and comparison applies equally to other concepts, such as morbidity and even mortality measures. Morbidity measures, for example, have been subject to different notification practices during different periods and in different countries. For this reason, data so collected or analysed may have limited generalisability. Death certificates are similarly ambiguous sources of data. The issuing of death certificates is an unsupervised, often unconsidered, frequently cursory activity carried out by doctors who consider the job 'routine' (Bloor 1991).

There has also been a history of criticism of existing statistical records, particularly government collections. Wigglesworth (1985) and Jenkins and others (1992) employ Australian examples in describing the inaccuracy of government collections. The latter issue highlights the problem of inherited methodological errors, while the example of death certification illustrates the problem of artificially categorising and reifying processes that are ambiguous and especially prone to human error.

Some concerns extend even to the very statistics used to work up a basic data set. Thus, there are concerns — as there always are surrounding favoured forms of measurement — about the statistics to use in secondary analysis. Several researchers have pointed to problems regarding the inappropriate comparison of incidence and prevalence data (Flanders & O'Brien 1989); the less than ideal use of Standardised Mortality Ratios (SMRs) and Gini coefficients (Carr-Hill 1990); the use of 'standard analytic approaches' that ignore complex patterns or interactions 'inherent in causal processes' (Dean et al. 1995).

There have been questions about the validity of operationalising health concerns around mortality data when there are any number of other ways to assess the health of a population. Is health status best indicated by death rates? Is lifestyle — as a complex and interacting set of physical, environmental and social factors — best operationalised around single variables such as smoking or nutritional intake? (Bloor 1991). Secondary analysis may, in this way, decontextualise the meanings of behaviour, thereby severely eroding the credibility and validity of any statements concerning 'risk' factors.

> **Disadvantages of secondary analysis of statistics**
> - Inherited methodological errors can distort analysis.
> - Generalisability is limited.
> - It artificially categorises processes that are ambiguous and changing.
> - It can decontextualise behaviour and its meaning.

Apart from the secondary analysis of statistics, further problems arise when we try to analyse narrative data, in the form of personal documents (letters, diaries, and so on) and public documents (such as newspapers and annual reports). Documents may contain data that are not necessarily truthful. Not all personal diaries are 'bare-all' tales of daily activities and thoughts, and few, if any, annual reports are written in that way. Writers write for an audience (even if it is only themselves), and they adapt their writing accordingly. A letter to one's mother does not contain the same information as a letter to a lover. A company report may be written for shareholders, even shareholders that the writer anticipates will be hostile. University handbooks are public-relations documents as much as they are sources of factual information. Newspapers are written for particular publics or markets, not for everyone imaginable. Consequently representativeness and bias may be problems.

For historical documents, there can be an additional problem of authenticity. A document believed to be associated with a particular writer (or writers) may, in fact, have been written by someone else. Not all photos are what they seem. Furthermore, data may be incomplete. The bulk of the public records of governments or private companies have been destroyed. Very few personal documents — even of famous people — manage to survive the personal vanity, guilt, or forgetfulness of their owners. And the ravages of time take a further toll on all documents.

Finally, understanding documents can be as frustrating as sorting through other people's statistics. Writing may be illegible. Attempts to understand the intended meaning, given the different meanings of words in certain historical periods or different cultural contexts, may be perilous. Personal codes or esoteric acronyms may further complicate your analysis.

> **Disadvantages of secondary analysis of narrative data**
> - Problems of representativeness and bias can distort analysis.
> - It is sometimes difficult to establish authenticity.
> - It is difficult to understand the meaning of some documents, especially out of context.
> - Sources are often incomplete.

The problems we have identified are not the 'death knell' of secondary analysis, as some would believe. They are important problems to bear in mind, but they are neither fatal nor insurmountable. Most research has 'limited generalisability', and often this is intentional. The limits of research findings are often readily admitted by those who conduct the analyses, and they can be seen as providing impetus for further work on a particular sample, or to adapt or test the findings on other populations.

The charge that secondary analysis artificially categorises processes that are ambiguous can be similarly overemphasised. Most, if not all, research categorises aspects of life — physiology, social circumstances, or class — that are ambiguous or changing. Photographs do this to life, but no one mistakes these photos for life itself. Representation is not invalid; no one claims that it is actually the thing it represents. Instead representation gives us indications of, or clues to, the often obscure or complex processes that underlie 'reality'.

It is true that sometimes secondary analysis can decontextualise meanings and behaviours, but so too can interviews, surveys, or observational work. The important theoretical issue to grasp is not that secondary analysis is particularly prone to this problem, because it is not, but that findings are rarely described without critical or informed discussion of them. Within that discussion, researchers describe, speculate, or theorise about the limits of their findings through critical interaction with other work and literature in the area. Some methods may decontextualise, but findings can still be rescued by contextualising the limits of the findings.

And, of course, the problem of identifying behaviour and meanings that are out of context can be addressed by designing studies that employ multiple methods. The use of single methods is frequently the offending feature, rather than a particular method in itself. Combining methods permits us to check findings, cross-validating the results of one method with those of another. This is also a powerful check on the hazards of inheriting methodological errors.

In addressing problems in using narrative data, it is important to be familiar with the secondary literature on the relevant subject. Rarely will one analyse the personal documents of certain individuals or people without also researching the history or sociology of those people, or the times or context in which a particular person lived or worked. For instance, one would not perform content-analysis on articles about Chinese alternative medicine in the *Journal of the American Medical Association* without also understanding the history and sociology of American medicine, particularly its professional attitudes to alternative models of medical cosmology.

As with secondary statistical data, it is important, if at all possible, that secondary analysis of narrative data be just one of a range of approaches to a particular issue, rather than the only approach. Cross-checking the data with *other methods* or with *other sources* is an important practice in all secondary analysis.

Some practical principles

The statistical procedures we might choose to perform on any given set of data will obviously depend on the type of data and the questions we bring to those data. In this respect, there is almost a limitless range of possibilities. If we are competent in this area, it will be the sources of data that will first interest us rather than the details of statistical procedures, which we might use later. There are four broad potential sources of data.

The first of these is, of course, *government sources*. Many university libraries have a government publication section in which census figures and the research from departments of health, immigration, welfare, education, or agriculture may be found. In Australia, these are usually Australian Government Publishing Service (AGPS) publications or Australian Bureau of Statistics (ABS) publications. In the United Kingdom, see the *HMSO Annual Catalogues*, and in the USA, the *Monthly Catalog of United States Government Publications*. There should also be some kind of guide to these sources published either by the relevant government publisher, the national library association, or perhaps even the university library itself (usually in the form of a self-published broadsheet or catalogue reference system).

For more recent and unpublished data sources, one can always phone the relevant department and enquire about current data-collection projects. In Australia, it often takes a long time to analyse data because of staff shortages, and sometimes, in these cases, departments will welcome offers of assistance in return for some rights to publish part of that analysis.

Theses or *dissertations* are also not to be overlooked as potential sources of secondary analysis. Thousands of theses are lodged every year that are never published, sometimes because publishers feel that their style or content does not reflect current tastes in book publishing or the dictates of the market. This is an area of hidden data sources that may well be worth searching *before* embarking on your own original work. Data in these areas will not necessarily turn up in standard computer searches of literature. A search through *Dissertations Abstracts International* may be especially useful here.

The *national data archive* is also worth an enquiry. These archives often contain repositories of data sets that are of no further interest to the people who compiled them. Polling agencies such as Gallup or newspaper surveys also frequently deposit their data sets in such archives. In the Australian archive (the Social Science Data Archive in Canberra), there is a diverse range of data sets from different studies. There are studies of teachers' attitudes, women in the public service, health knowledge and drug-use among high school students, Vietnamese refugees, blood pressure studies, and even the role of pharmacists in patient counselling. The annual guide to these sets is worth consulting.

Finally, there are the various *directories of information* published by private authors, usually librarians, which provide a guide to information and records. One of the many British guides (Codlin 1990) provides lists of five and a half thousand organisations that make information available on issues as diverse as AIDS and Bach. The National Society of Archives is also worth consulting for numerical and non-numerical data sources. (In Australia, see Burnstein et al. 1992; or in the USA, see, for example, National Historical Publications and Records Commission 1988).

In connection with archives, do not neglect the possible sources of data to be found in *registries*: births, deaths, and marriages, but also the active records of companies and professional organisations. The Australian Medical Association or the National Farmers Federation (NFF) are just two examples of frequently overlooked data sources for the public health researcher.

There are also a number of important researcher guides to registries, archives, and libraries, and detailed discussions of their holdings. In the same vein, there are books on 'unobtrusive research', 'secondary analysis', 'life history' and 'personal documents'. All these subjects are particularly relevant to analysis of letters, *vox populi* (qualitative interview data), diaries, and oral history. We recommend some of these key references at the end of the chapter.

Data sources for the secondary analyst
- government publications
- government departments
- theses and dissertations
- archives (all sorts, but especially data archives for numerical data)
- libraries (especially for narrative data)
- registries
- national directories of information
- professional associations
- company records

When dealing with narrative data sources, you may not necessarily want to analyse that material statistically. Often you will need to analyse the data much as a humanities or social science scholar would. In this sense you will be applying the skills of content, thematic, or semiotic analysis — common analytic styles in these discipline areas. The public health researcher who wishes to analyse narrative data will also need to be familiar with these styles of analysis.

The practice of *content-analysis* assumes that you know what you wish to search for in the narrative material. You may, for example, wish to note how many times death is discussed in a personal diary or set of letters. You might also wish to know any details that appear in those records about diet. You will then trawl the record with those particular categories (and perhaps others) in mind. In other words, you *decide the categories that you wish to search for before the actual search.* Traditional content-analysis is selecting *a priori* the categories that *you*, as researcher, believe are important. The emphasis is on *your* categories and the *frequency* of their occurrence.

In *thematic analysis*, the material (the letters, the diary, or the company minutes, for example) is searched for *themes that emerge as being important to the participants or writer.* It is the writer's or participant's point of view that is important in discerning these themes. The themes that emerge then become the categories of the subsequent analysis. As with content-analysis, the themes may be clustered together to form overriding themes, or the original themes may contain sub-themes that support the larger themes. The sub-themes are evidence for the construction or observation of the larger themes. However, mere frequency does not necessarily indicate the importance of an identified theme. The *position* of the idea in the narrative may be more important. For example, sexism may not be very evident in the numerous stories and sections of a daily newspaper. However, the little evidence of sexism that there is may consistently appear on the front page, or on the first few pages, shedding light on the importance of these messages for the newspaper concerned. In this case, it is not the frequency but the strategic position of the idea that is telling or evidential.

Semiotic analysis goes further than simply analysing the manifest themes. The researcher asks questions to deepen the data-analysis: What is missing here? What is not being said or written, and why? Why are certain words or phrases chosen by the writer and not others? What is the possible significance of those choices and preferences?

As you might have surmised from these descriptions, content-analysis is concerned with measurement and is closely aligned with the positivist preference for hypothesis-testing. Evidence and reliability are strong for this style of analysis, but generalisations can be restrained and limited. Thematic analysis (common in qualitative work) is a little more subjective but can, nonetheless, be subject to sound inter-rater corroboration. Its evidence can be strong and its generalisations more reflective of other people's meanings. Semiotic analysis is the art of literary and social theorists, and represents the opposite methodological position of positivism. Similar to the legal profession, it celebrates the case and the precedent, highlights the importance of persuasion based on appealing to others' experience, and assumes that appearances are rarely what they seem.

Accordingly, the semiotic analyst would argue that there are many insights that the obvious probing of positivism is incapable of accessing. We do not have enough space to further explore these analytic styles, but the recommended reading at the end of this chapter suggests some important references for those who are interested.

Analytical strategies for narrative data

1 Content-analysis:
- searches for *a priori* categories
- focuses on frequency and researchers' categories.

2 Thematic analysis:
- identifies emergent categories
- privileges the authorial view of a category's importance.

3 Semiotic analysis:
- identifies emergent and missing categories
- takes a critical view of authorial categories.

Ethics: not a secondary consideration

We should not make the mistake of thinking that, just because there are no respondents to whom we can relate in secondary analysis, there are few ethical concerns relevant to this type of work; nothing could be further from the truth. There are just as many ethical problems involved in working with other people's data — numerical or narrative — as there are in obtaining data directly from subjects or respondents.

The first issue is still one of consent. Ethically (if not legally), data belong to someone. Except in rare instances — for example, published government statistics — the public health researcher should seek permission to use most data from archives, theses, or companies. Furthermore, acknowledgment or even co-authorship may be a part of this ethical consideration, depending on how unique the existing data are or how important they are to one's 'new' contribution. This issue will need to be reviewed very carefully. As always, it is worth discussing this with others to gain a more social view of how this issue might be viewed by peers.

Access to some archives or data may be restricted, as is sometimes the case with active files in registries, for example. There is sometimes a temptation to downplay one's interest in, or plans for, the data so as not unduly to interest or concern the owners or minders of that data. This is misrepresenting your role and possible aims, and is to be avoided. Informed consent to use data requires that the original 'owner' of the data be informed of all intentions to analyse and publish those data. In any case, if your intentions are not clear at the outset, and a decision to publish is made later on, permission should be sought again. Permission to use data should not be conveniently conflated with permission to publish; *both* should be obtained if both are desired at any point in the research. When seeking permission to publish, it may be relevant to explore issues of copyright. Personal documents, company records, or large extracts from published accounts may fall into this category.

Confidentiality is also an ethical concern, and this applies especially to narrative data. Authors of letters or diaries may be dead, but the contents may still affect living relatives or copyright-owners. Once again, permission to study the diaries is not the same as permission to publish extracts or to publicly reveal information contained therein.

It is also important to remember that the issue of harm is not restricted to randomised control trials or observational studies. Fook (1991), for example, performed a content-analysis of descriptions of university social work courses that appeared in university handbooks. She was interested in studying the impact of feminist and socialist thinking on these courses. However, no university was named in the study. Such results, whatever the outcome or conclusions, could influence student enrolments adversely. In turn, this can have negative consequences for contracted staff. We must always consider the potential of results to cause unintentional harm.

Finally, cheating is also an important issue to identify. Of particular importance is the problem of plagiarism. Be careful not to steal data. When using tracts of commentary or ideas from other sources, always acknowledge these in a citation. Because some data can come from obscure and difficult sources, it is sometimes difficult to recheck these data. The onus is always on the researcher to represent these data with care and honesty.

Recommended reading

Carr-Hill, R. 1990, 'The Measurement of Inequities in Health: Lessons from the British Experience', *Social Science and Medicine*, vol. 31, no. 3, pp. 393–404.

Dale, A., Arber, S., & Proctor, M. 1986, *Doing Secondary Analysis*, George Allen & Unwin, London.

Kellehear, A. 1993, *The Unobtrusive Researcher: A Guide to Methods*, Allen & Unwin, Sydney.

For an introductory overview of content, thematic, and semiotic styles of analysis, see chapters 2 and 3.

Maher, C. & Burke, T. 1991, *Informed Decision Making*, Longman Cheshire, Melbourne.

See chapters 1–3 especially.

Manning, P.K. 1987, *Semiotics and Fieldwork*, Sage, Beverly Hills, Calif.

Miles, M.B. & Huberman, A.M. 1984, *Qualitative Data Analysis*, Sage, Beverly Hills, Calif.

Plummer, K. 1983, *Documents of Life*, George Allen & Unwin, London.

Stewart, D. 1984, *Secondary Research: Information Sources and Methods*, Sage, Beverly Hills, Calif.

Weber, R.P. 1990, *Basic Content Analysis*, Sage, Newbury Park, Calif.

CHAPTER 10

Meta-analysis

Imagine twenty or thirty, or even a hundred, different studies of health risks associated with a particular treatment intervention. Few of these studies agree with one another, and more than a few contradict the conclusions of the majority. Imagine further, if you can, the idea of sweeping all these individual papers together and integrating their findings to develop a fresh numerical assessment and overview of them all. While it is not necessarily a narrative review of the literature, this 'analysis of analyses' (Glass 1976) is commonly a statistical reassessment of the heterogeneous trends in other people's studies. This is 'meta-analysis' — a state-of-the-art review of all the available data on a particular subject.

Because meta-analysis is a *systematic* review of all available data in an area, there has been an attempt to create formal criteria for the inclusion of studies. The purpose of these criteria is to avoid the subjectively biased selection that can occur in traditional literature reviews. Meta-analysts also attempt to assess the influence of study design on the end results of a range of individual studies. Finally, in the overall interpretation of findings in an area, meta-analysts attempt to factor out or control their own prejudices or opinions in the weightings given to particular studies (Wolf 1986).

Olkin (1995) provides some brief historical notes about meta-analysis. In 1904 Karl Pearson analysed five studies of the effectiveness of inoculation on enteric fever. Despite this early medical interest, Olkin observes that agriculture was the primary catalyst for the development of this style of re-analysis during the 1930s and 1940s. Industrial groups also showed some interest in this method. However, interest was dormant during the 1950s and 1960s, and the method did not re-emerge until Glass used the approach in educational research in 1976.

Chalmers and Haynes (1994) observed that before 1982 a search of the Medline (a library search tool that abstracts all medical journal articles published) might reveal as little as one meta-analysis a year. Between 1982 and 1985, this figure rose to something like fifteen a year. In 1992, however, a search of Medline using the newly established search term 'meta-analysis' yielded over 500 citations.

The current interest in meta-analysis as a method is so great that the production of a CD-ROM database has recently been undertaken. The enormous task of reviewing the existing data in medical research literature, such as it is, has begun (see the Cochrane Database of Systematic Reviews; and Sackett & Oxman 1994). Journals such as the *Lancet*, the *British Medical Journal* and the *Annals of Internal Medicine* regularly carry reviews, debates, and editorials dealing with this latest of methods in public health research.

Some examples

The interested reader can now choose from literally thousands of examples of meta-analysis. F.R. Rosendaal (1994) observes that there are three types of meta-analyses: those that aim for a higher statistical power (that is, lower p-values, which indicate higher probability) than may have been achieved by other studies; those that aim to achieve the best risk estimate from a diverse and sometimes conflicting set of studies (a kind of averaging exercise that might reveal some underlying, invariant relation) (Hunter et al. 1982); and those that attempt to answer questions that the original studies were not designed to answer. Whatever the type, the meta-analytic approach is now clearly on the ascendant in public health. A scattered overview of the topics addressed by meta-analyses shows the diversity of interests to which this method is currently being applied.

There are meta-analyses on the impact of neuroleptic medication on tardive dyskinesia (Morgenstern et al. 1987); the dependence potential of short half-life Benzodiazepines (Hallfors & Saxe 1993); oral contraceptives and the risk of gall-bladder disease (Thijs & Knipschild 1993); chlorination and cancer (Morris et al. 1992); and the validity of self-reports of smoking (Patrick et al. 1994). There are other meta-analyses on the effectiveness of drug-abuse resistance education programs (Ennett et al. 1994); condom-effectiveness in reducing sexually transmitted HIV (Weller 1993; Warner & Hatcher 1994); help-seeking behaviour and breast cancer symptoms (Facione 1993); potential harm and benefits from screening for colorectal cancer (Towler et al. 1995); and estimated rates of unaided smoking cessation (Baillie et al. 1995).

Grady and others (1992) reviewed the risks and benefits of hormone therapy for asymptomatic menopausal women who are considering long-term hormone replacement therapy for the prevention of disease and to prolong life. They reviewed all English-language studies that have appeared since 1970. Employing statistical methods to create an overall estimate of relative risks, they compared length of hormone intake with type of hormone and incidence of certain diseases, particularly endometrial cancer, breast cancer, coronary heart disease, hip fracture, and stroke.

The results of these reviews have often had important implications for clinical and academic work in their respective areas. Glasziou and Mackerras (1993), for example, examined twenty controlled trials (from 1969 to 1992) to assess the effectiveness of vitamin A supplementation on morbidity and mortality rates from infectious diseases. They found that adequate sources of vitamin A, from diet or supplements, did indeed play a major role in lowering morbidity and mortality rates, especially in developing countries. In developed countries, supplementation had its uses too, particularly in preventing life-threatening infections such as measles.

Stewart and others (1995) conducted a meta-analysis of twenty-four population-based studies 'which contributed a total of 168 gender and age specific estimates of migraine prevalence' (p. 269). They found a remarkable level of stability in these estimates.

Mumford and others (1982) provided another quantitative review of thirty-four controlled studies that assessed the effect of 'psychological intervention' in people recovering from surgery or heart attacks. They found that, compared with groups that did not receive even modest interventions, groups that did receive these attentions experienced less post-operative complications and less anxiety, and went home earlier. This study highlights one of the truly interesting and valuable contributions of meta-analyses: it is often in areas in which the findings are somewhat equivocal — or in which findings are spread widely over an area that is largely interdisciplinary — that a careful meta-analysis and review paper is able to shed some valuable light.

Another positive example of this can be seen in Levin's (1994) study of the relationship between religion and health. He asked three intriguing and important questions of that relationship: Is there an association? Is it valid? Is it causal? In a cross between a review of the literature and conventional meta-analysis, Levin examined the results of a large number of diverse studies and review papers on this topic. Included in his analysis was a review of over 250 empirical studies dating back to the nineteenth century. Carefully sifting through this literature, Levin observed that an association between religion (variously defined) and health (defined according to both morbidity and mortality data) did exist. In determining the validity of the finding, Levin argues that the diversity and volume of these studies and their designs may actually be a factor working to the 'advantage of validity'. As for whether 'religion' may be a confounding variable — that is, a variable disguising a more specific influence such as dietary regimes or protective psychosocial effects — Levin cautions against reductionism.

While the influence of psychosocial factors can generally be understood in terms of biological processes or mechanisms, this does not imply that psychosocial variables are not meaningfully related to health. For example, while there is greater mortality among lonely widows and single men, it is hardly sufficient to say that this is fully explained by psycho-neuro-immunological factors, even though the process of mortality is reducible to certain physiological and biochemical events. Granting explanatory primacy to one particular level of the human system (cultural, social, psychological, organ systems, cellular, or molecular, for example) is arbitrary; human biology itself is 'explained' by the activity of molecules, and ultimately, to paraphrase Democritus, everything is just atoms and empty space. Yet no one would suggest that research in subatomic physics will yield the best approach for improving the life expectancy of lonely or bereaved people (Levin 1994: 1477).

Levin's answer to the final question of causality is a reflective 'maybe'. In terms of consistency, plausibility, and coherence of the data, causality seems likely. But in terms of the paucity of experimental designs and overall strength of data, one cannot be sure. Too few epidemiological studies have been designed to explore these issues, and no single quantitative meta-analysis of all the hundreds of studies has been undertaken to date. Notwithstanding, the data up until now suggest intriguing and tantalising promise for, if not one, then several meta-analyses focusing on different aspects of religion and health.

Advantages and disadvantages

Levin's study highlights two important and positive observations about meta-analysis. First meta-analyses are not necessarily just statistical summaries and combinations of information, although this is a dominant interpretation of the Cochrane Collaboration. However, as Liberati (1995: 82) rightly notes, those strategies may not always be possible or warranted by an area: 'It is misleading to equate meta-analysis, or systematic review for that matter, to a pure statistical technique or approach'. In this connection, we can understand meta-analysis as part of the formal scientific practice of assessment and overview of a particular area. And although this approach has become increasingly quantitative in the last ten years or so, its technical achievements and contribution are not to be wholly identified with that statistical dominance.

Second, as Spitzer (1995) noted in his keynote address at the Potsdam Conference on Meta-analysis, few of the 'big' questions about major suffering can be answered by a single study or even a few studies considered together. And yet, as Spitzer observes, there is a need — sometimes an urgent need — to address some of these unresolved questions, even if it only involves trawling old data to look for new directions in which we might turn for an answer.

These points are also two of the major advantages of employing meta-analysis as a method, but they are not the only advantages. Victor (1995) also remarks that meta-analyses are advantageous when an urgent decision needs to be made, but a lack of time renders the conduct of a new trial impossible. Research on the safety of drugs also makes meta-analysis a particularly relevant procedure because the exclusion of any study on side-effects, for example, is unwise.

Finally, meta-analysis can be a useful way of panning back and gaining an overview of an area in which most of the studies are inconclusive because the effects are small, or contradictory, or the power of individual studies is limited. In this context, meta-analyses can provide methodological 'best practice' evaluation of the dominant research designs in the area. As Spitzer (1995: 7) warns, 'Results of meta-analysis can only be interpreted if existing heterogeneities can be adequately explained by methodological heterogeneities'. In other words, a final advantage of meta-analyses is their contribution to assessing the quality of clinical trials and medical literature in general (Liberati 1995). More than simply a literature review, the *predefined inclusion criteria and systematic nature* of meta-analysis encourage fairer and more reliable assessments of the methods and results in an area.

Advantages of meta-analysis

Meta-analyses are able to provide:
- the ability to identify an invariant finding in a diverse array of similarly designed studies
- systematic assessment and overview of findings in an area
- an ability to address larger research questions
- an alternative method when others are not possible (for example, because of time or population constraints)
- methodological assessments of current research designs.

Meta-analysis has been a controversial method. It has aroused much bitter, and at times cynical, debate. For some people, the randomised control trial remains the gold standard of research, and meta-analysis (indeed any non–randomised control trial approach) is considered 'poor science'. Other people who are frustrated by the one-eyed, narrow, some say 'decontextualised' approach of single studies have hailed meta-analysis as a necessary method because it enables the researcher to rise above the problem of science's information explosion. Not only can meta-analysis provide a state-of-the-art overview and review of methods and results in an area, but it can also be a basis for justifying and informing new work or discouraging fruitless repetition.

Nevertheless, the following problems are regularly discussed and debated in the literature. First, some writers have argued that meta-analysis camouflages whole groups of studies with fancy statistics. The significance of these studies may be mediocre or weak, but this is difficult to assess because of the complexity of the retrospective application of esoteric numerical procedures. This leads to the charge that meta-analysis is unnecessarily obscure.

Second, and related to this anxiety about the rigour of meta-analytic studies, is the accusation that these approaches fall prey to the 'file drawer problem' (also known as 'publication bias') (Last 1995). This phrase suggests that there will always be a quantity of studies that have insignificant findings, and therefore these studies will not find their way to publication — they are simply dropped into the office file system never to see the light of day. Those collected studies that are published and assessed as a group, by simple process of being drawn together for the purposes of summary, will exaggerate the statistical significance in any chosen area because negative cases are excluded. This is a charge of bias.

Linked to this concern about bias is the further related issue of how misleading this kind of approach can be. Stewart and Parmar (1993), for example, compared meta-analysis of literature (MAL) with meta-analysis of individual patient data (MAP) and found that MAL did exaggerate conclusions in an examination of cisplatin therapy in ovarian cancer. The MAL gave results of greater statistical significance ($p = 0.027$ versus $p = 0.30$) and an estimate of absolute treatment effect three times as large as MAP (7.5 per cent versus 2.5 per cent). Stewart and Palmer have not been the only ones to raise this concern about misleading results using this method (see also Egger & Smith 1995; Bailar 1995).

Third, meta-analysis can be used (or, as Victor (1995)puts it, 'misused') as a way of avoiding the hard work of actually conducting one's own study or set of studies. This idea has led to charges of intellectual or methodological laziness. This can also encourage other writers and workers to submit small studies with weak levels of significance. Authors and editors might rationalise their submission and subsequent acceptance in journals on the basis that some meta-analysis will come along some day and rescue these results through their incorporation into some larger statistical or theoretical picture. Some have called these tendencies an encouragement to second-rate research (Victor 1995).

Fourth, one of the strengths of meta-analysis is its ability to provide *systematic* reviews of an area. This claim to thoroughness is believed to be a major advance over single trials or subjective overviews of selected studies. Nevertheless, if this ability to be systematic were compromised (by limitations in current search technologies, for example), this might also be a significant criticism and limitation of the method, something to be viewed as an important barrier to best practice.

In fact, there is already some suggestion that this problem does exist. Dickersin and others (1994) decided to examine the sensitivity and precision of Medline search abilities in identifying studies for meta-analysis.

The 'gold standard' they used as a criterion was all randomised control trials known to them in ophthalmology in 1988. They found that they were able to turn up 51 per cent of *all* studies — both those indexed in Medline and those not in Medline. But even had they confined themselves to those within the Medline database, the figure only manages to rise to 76 per cent. This leads to the charge that the systematic reviews boasted by meta-analysis may be less than systematic.

Finally, of course, there are the more technical problems. Some regressions are non-linear but are discussed as if they were; some samples and some data-collection instruments are of a dubious nature. For example, Eysenck (1994) examined passive-smoking studies that contain significant sub-samples of casual or ex-smokers, thereby casting doubt upon the reliability and validity of rates of lung cancer among 'non-smokers'. In the same review he discusses several psychometric instruments that have questionable reliability and validity, and identifies some that have been employed in well-known meta-analyses. Also, heterogeneity is too commonly explained by authors of meta-analyses as simply reflecting heterogeneity in target populations or treatments. This may not be true. The sources of heterogeneity need examination, for they may be due to irregularities in the scientific or clinical designs of the original studies.

Disadvantages of meta-analysis

Meta-analyses may be:
- obscure
- biased and misleading
- an encouragement to laziness and lack of rigour
- ironically unsystematic
- technically unreliable or, worse, invalid.

How serious are these charges? The short answer is 'not very'. Much of the criticism can be likened to giving the 'new kid on the block' a hard time. Established scientific methods, like old established networks, are the stuff of exclusive neighbourhoods. However, some of the criticism is not without substance. Let us first address criticism that seems to represent a general and amorphous resistance to meta-analysis. Although much of this criticism is valid, it cannot be said to apply only to meta-analysis. If, as is commonly the case, this is not frankly admitted, the criticism then appears to single the method out, perhaps to reject or isolate it unfairly.

The charge of obscurity is an old one and is frequently applied to any set of methods or procedures with which the reader is unfamiliar. In fact, this is a charge often levelled at social science studies by medical researchers and vice versa. Indeed, this is a common complaint in relation to all statistics, hence the saying 'Lies, damn lies and statistics'. Fancy statistics are not a unique or characterising feature of meta-analysis, any more than they are characteristic of randomised control trials, quality-of-life measures, or large scale epidemiological surveys. We should all be vigilant against mathematical or literary expressions that mitigate against clear understanding, irrespective of the difficulty of the idea or calculation.

The charge of bias is, once again, not unique to the problems of meta-analysis, and is a problem that must be guarded against in all studies. Sample-selection, poor data-collection instruments, or inappropriate use or interpretation of statistics are the stuff of debate — and very constructive debate — about all the main public health methods, their designs, and their conclusions. No one in any research culture seriously doubts this, and so we should be careful not to identify these problems exclusively with meta-analysis. For every poor example of meta-analysis, we can produce a similar example of a flawed randomised control trial, or of a meta-analysis that does not suffer from these problems. All methods are dogged by problematic users.

That meta-analysis encourages laziness in research is an odd charge, for laziness — like beauty and the positive attributes of friends — is clearly in the eye of the beholder. Who is to say that meta-analysis is a lazy person's way of escaping from the 'hard work' of a proper trial? Perhaps the conducting of yet another trial indicates that some researchers, locked into comfortable old habits, are resisting the 'hard work' of sifting through possibly hundreds of past trials to determine whether another is worth their effort or their subject's discomfort.

It has become fashionable to sneer at weak levels of significance, but one need only remind readers that levels of significance are called that because they are that: significant. If low levels are not respectable, why bother to record them? If there is any significant methodological error, low levels of significance may be subject to a certain erosion of confidence, but this reflects a problem with study selection and not statistics. We will address that problem below.

Finally, there is the charge that systematic reviews may be less than systematic. Of course, this is concerning, but it is hardly a new problem or one confined, once again, to meta-analysis. This is a potential criticism of *all* studies that sample in any way, whether this sampling is of literature or of human populations. We need to examine the problem on a case-by-case basis and not condemn particular methods as a whole because these problems of sampling are found among them. We repeat: these are user problems, and little evidence has surfaced to date to show that meta-analysis is particularly prone to this widely relevant problem.

In connection with being less than systematic, Liberati (1995: 85) usefully reminds us that 'before killing systematic reviews in medicine one should never forget what is the only available alternative to them, i.e. the unsystematic, implicit, qualitative review'.

To redress some of the relevant criticism of meta-analysis, several useful and thoughtful suggestions have been made by workers experienced in the area. Egger and Smith (1995) suggest that more research into the factors associated with misleading meta-analyses should be undertaken to help us discover which problems are clearly specific to that method and which are commonly shared problems. There is also a need to carefully scrutinise all studies that are used in any meta-analysis, noting their particular problems and discussing these explicitly. In particular, they suggest that a register of all trials could be established so that negative studies do not disappear from view and may be factored into future assessments in any particular area. Compiling such a register, however, is one enormous task. Wachter (1988) has also suggested that statistical methods of maximum likelihood estimation be pressed into service for this particular problem. Egger and Smith also contend that all meta-analyses based on small trials should be distrusted. They argue that several 'medium'-sized trials need to be included before one can feel confidence in any particular meta-analysis. Finally, Bailar (1995: 156) warns that meta-analyses should never be seen to replace the traditional literature review, for whatever the problems of traditional reviews, they are nevertheless able to 'do far more than estimate parameters and the additions are critical to the progress of science'.

At the end of the day, science is the domain of creative ideas and of the unnoticed connections between them; it is not simply about arguments over estimates. Meta-analysts should be very familiar with the primary literature they are reviewing. Statistical prowess alone, without clinical or academic familiarity, is not adequate to the task of successful and thorough meta-analysis. Equipped with this sensible advice, how might one begin?

Some practical principles

It is not the purpose of this section to go into the statistical intricacies of meta-analysis. This is an area of such incredible diversity that Feinstein (1995: 74) remarked that someone perhaps ought to do a meta-analysis of this diversity to gain some semblance of agreement about what the best statistical operations are for this purpose. Those interested in these numerical issues might first look at Hedges and Olkin (1985), Hunter and others (1982), or Wolf (1986) in the recommended reading at the end of this chapter. Feinstein's critical article (1995), in which he admirably plays the devil's advocate, should also be read.

The basic principles for beginning any meta-analysis are summarised in a variety of journals and books, but the advice of Macarthur and others (1995), and of Clarke and Stewart (1994), is among the simplest and clearest. The first requirement is that researchers should formulate their research question as precisely as possible. They should then attempt to develop criteria or protocols according to which studies will and will not be included in the meta-analysis. Criteria for the evaluation of methodological quality also need to be developed, as well as some way of generally assessing which studies are compatible or 'combinable' with the research objectives or questions. At this stage, the quality of the data needs to be evaluated. The researcher combs the literature, choosing studies with comparable interventions and outcomes. Differences in patient samples, protocols, or confounding variables need to be closely examined. Any inclusion of data from different samples, interventions, or outcomes needs careful justification. As Goodman (1991) wryly observes in his discussion of these points, meta-analysis is not an excuse to throw absolutely everything and anything together. When the criteria have been determined, the data are then extracted and analysed, with calculations made for the summary effect if this is appropriate.

In addition to these suggestions, Clarke and Stewart (1994) make three other useful suggestions, which complement those of Macarthur and his colleagues. In searching for studies to include in your meta-analysis, you should make an attempt to contact all the authors of those studies (see, for example, Pocock, Smith, & Baghurst 1994). This step can lead to valuable additional information, which will minimise bias in the meta-analysis being developed. It may, for example, lead to the identification of studies not unearthed through Medline searches or your net of library-based searches. It may also reveal studies not previously published and their whereabouts.

When analysing the data, it is important to look carefully at all randomised *and* non-randomised participants, since this sampling can lead to significant bias in later calculations. Some patients are randomised but are not included in a study because they are later found to be ineligible for one reason or another. Other participants are not randomised but are included in the study because they represent an earlier non-randomised part of the larger study. If this information is not obvious from the publication, then it might also be obtained from correspondence or telephone calls to the original trialists.

But you should not think that all bias has been minimised by carefully checking for unknown or overlooked studies, and by scrutinising the sample selection/inclusion processes. Feinstein reminds us that bias can

---

To conduct a meta-analysis, you will need to:

1 precisely formulate your research objectives or questions
2 develop criteria for
   - the inclusion and exclusion of studies
   - evaluating the methodologies
   - assessing 'combinabilty'
   - assessing the quality of data
3 search and retrieve studies (that is, through a library search and through other possible means), making an attempt to contact the authors of any studies you wish to use
4 extract and analyse the data, taking both randomised and non-randomised participants into consideration and, if possible, checking all individual patient data
5 make conclusions regarding a treatment's performance or the detection of an outcome, being careful to eliminate any bias.

---

also creep in at the level of assessing a treatment's performance and detecting an outcome, and these factors need to be considered in any final discussion of the meta-analysis. Finally, if possible, all individual patient data should be checked, if only for error and the occasional fraud.

Ethical matters

Ethical matters are seldom discussed by meta-analysts, and just as disturbingly, they rarely find their way into the many debates and discussions about this new method to be found in journals. An exception is an article by Rosendaal (1994), which argues that meta-analysis is not original work but simply the reworking of others' original work. Simply summarising, recalculating, and then summarising again, meta-analysts make their assessments on the back of other people's work. This procedure, he argues, is akin to plagiarism. To counter this 'unfairness', he believes that meta-analysts must give due credit to the original authors through co-authorship of any subsequent work based on their earlier data or findings.

Cook and Guyatt (1994), in a paper that followed Rosendaal's, contend that this view is nonsense because of what, they argue, is Rosendaal's ridiculous attempt to stratify the value and worth of other people's research. Indeed, Rosendaal does tend to confuse or over-identify original research with primary or empirical research, and he does not accord secondary, historical, or review work the originality it demonstrates by making connections that have not been noticed before. Rosendaal seems to believe that it is the data themselves, rather than their interpretation, that are the principle component of originality — a quaint, if not naïve, view of science. Furthermore, he fails to understand that, one way or another, all work is built on the work of others. Indeed, his ethical injunction to invite all authors connected in some way to the research to co-author 'new' work would ensure that the main part of any article would be the list of its 'authors'.

But in dismissing Rosendaal's concerns about ethics too quickly, Cook and Guyatt themselves overreact and fail to discuss the issue of ethics at all. As we have seen in earlier chapters on other methods, ethical matters are important because they are concerned with discussing the most responsible way of conducting research — the responsibility, in this case, being to colleagues and the wider community.

When using the work of others, the onus is on the meta-analyst always to use the work conservatively and with great respect for the limitations of the data. For example, data may be handled uncritically: 'good' randomised control trials are sometimes lumped together with 'poor' ones, without weighted codes being used to accommodate differences in the calculations. The criteria for assessing the meta-analysis's sources of heterogeneity need to be taken very seriously. It is important to ensure that poor methods — both in one's own analysis and in other people's — do not translate into erroneous conclusions with both social and ethical implications. In this way, good ethics can be equated with good science.

Additionally, when using unpublished case material, the meta-analyst needs to ensure confidentiality of the case-record material. Those colleagues who have entrusted you with these data should not be misled, and you should undertake not to use the data for any *additional* purpose without the permission of the original researchers. Clarke and Stewart (1994) argue that, if any published papers do, in fact, use the data for permitted additional purposes, then the original authors could expect to be included as co-authors of these subsequent analyses and publications. Similarly, these original trialists should be given the opportunity to comment on pre-publication drafts.

Feinstein (1995), citing earlier work by Meinert (1989), also warns that trialists who are contacted for further information, or who are encouraged to supply their original data sets in some form or another, are often being asked to produce work with no remuneration and little, if any, prospect of recognition. This issue needs to be taken into account when thinking about the possible benefits to one's study versus the costs to others in time and effort. It is an issue of fairness.

Another ethical problem is that meta-analyses give, or can give, a kind of finality to studies in a certain area. This means that a meta-analysis can unwittingly give the impression that its conclusions are the final verdict, yet trials in that area may not be over. This can, as Feinstein puts it, give the impression of 'winners' and 'losers' in an area of research. A potentially dangerous and misleading impression can be conveyed, particularly if results are premature or are prematurely released to the media. Not only may this be misleading, but it may also constitute a public and scientific nuisance. The pressure to use the media to increase public sympathy and to encourage government to fund certain areas has led to close relationships between researchers and the media. Whatever their benefits, researchers should be aware that even the most encouraging results can never entirely avoid the problem of being misleading, at least in an unfolding historical sense. In this context, then, the decision to use the media always has serious ethical implications requiring the careful attention and consideration of all researchers, meta-analysts or not.

Recommended reading

Eysenck, H.J. 1994, 'Meta-analysis and Its Problems', *British Medical Journal*, vol. 309, pp. 789–92.

Feinstein, A.R. 1995, 'Meta-analysis: Statistical Alchemy for the 21st Century', *Journal of Clinical Epidemiology*, vol. 48, no. 1, pp. 71–9.

This and the excellent Olkin article cited below are from the proceedings of the 1994 Potsdam International Consultation on Meta-analysis (Germany), which were published a special issue of the *Journal of Clinical Epidemiology*. Those wishing to read all the contributions are directed to volume 48, number 1, of that journal.

Glass, G., McGaw, B. & Smith, M. Lee 1981, *Meta-analysis in Social Research*, Sage, Beverly Hills, Calif.

The inventor of the term 'meta-analysis' (Glass) and his colleagues provide good advice on coding and measurement.

Hedges, L.V. & Olkin, I. 1985, *Statistical Methods for Meta-analysis*, Academic Press, New York.

The title speaks for itself.

Hunter, J., Schmidt, F., & Jackson, G. 1982, *Meta-analysis: Cumulating Research Findings across Studies*, Sage, Beverly Hills, Calif.

A good introduction to the statistics involved.

Louis, T.A., Fineberg, H.V., & Mosteller, F. 1985, 'Findings for Public Health from Meta-analyses', *Annual Review of Public Health*, vol. 6, pp. 1–20.

Olkin, I. 1995, 'Statistical and Theoretical Considerations in Meta-analysis', *Journal of Clinical Epidemiology*, vol. 48, no. 1, pp. 133–46.

Pettiti, D. 1994, *Meta-analysis, Decision-Analysis and Cost-Effective Analysis: Methods of Quantitative Synthesis in Medicine*, Oxford University Press, New York.

A good overview of the area with nice 'how-to' sections.

Wachter, K. & Straf, M. 1990 (eds), *The Future of Meta-analysis*, Russell Sage Foundation, New York.

A good overview with case studies.

Wolf, F. 1986, *Meta-analysis: Quantitative Methods for Research Systems*, Sage, Beverly Hills, Calif.

Another guide to the appropriate statistics to use in meta-analysis.

CHAPTER 11

Qualitative Innovations

There are some of us working in public health who started our working lives in the laboratory. Sometimes, after a bad day in the field, we find ourselves longing for the security and control that laboratory researchers have over the material in their test tubes: it mostly stays put, and it does not talk back. But then we remember why we left. The real world throws up important public health problems that simply cannot be solved in the laboratory.

As Linus in the *Peanuts* cartoons knows, it takes courage to let go of a security blanket. It is equally hard for researchers to let go of the security of being able to control the 'objects' of their research. Some of us keep to experimental designs, despite the difficulty of trying to make our live 'subjects' behave in a properly experimental manner. These researchers do randomised control trials. Others give up the task of disciplining the research 'subject' altogether and instead discipline themselves to observe people in a structured and rigorous manner. These researchers do observational studies. The brave among us go so far as to ask people what they are doing, using a structured questionnaire, and we trust them (more or less) to tell us the truth. Here the method of choice is the questionnaire survey. The next stage in letting go of control is to ask people to tell us about their experiences in their own way. The in-depth interview is the result. Perhaps bravery becomes foolhardiness in those researchers who ask groups of people to talk freely about their experiences. They conduct focus group research.

So far, the methods described are all the subject of scholarly texts addressing methodological issues. If some of the methods are new to us, we at least know that other researchers have been using them, admittedly with varying degrees of success, for some time. But there are those among us who appear not to know when to stop — at least from the point of view of the Linus-type researchers. They find that they actually *like* the freedom of letting go of their security blankets. They are prepared to dispense with the tried and tested methods and go it alone. They are the innovators.

Innovators using qualitative methods usually fall into one (or even both) of two categories: they combine existing methods in a flexible manner or they push existing methods beyond the boundaries within which they are usually applied. Let us deal with each type in turn.

Combining methods is a bit like shining lights of various colours on a topic, shifting from one colour to the other, but with the final analysis synthesising the combined effect of what the different coloured lights have displayed. The big advantages of a compendium of methods are flexibility and the ability to probe a setting for any kind of material that would be useful and to collect it in the most rigorous manner. The problem here is that we may end up with too few data to do a proper analysis of any one approach. On the other hand, is that not exactly what happens when we conduct a series of inconclusive trials? As with trials, the answer is to use a method for synthesising the results to get an overall answer of increased power.

Innovators can also push the boundaries of personal interview studies and focus group studies. The definition of an interview can be extended, for instance, to include interviews done in an informal manner, on the run, or perhaps while researchers actually participate in the activity being studied. Or they might push the limits of the group interview to take in the whole of a community, with anything anybody says or does potentially being used as data. The line dividing the researcher and the research participant breaks down as the researcher starts behaving much like a study participant and vice versa.

As we move out of the laboratory into these uncharted waters, we lose control over the collection of data from our research 'subjects', but what also slips away from us is a clearly defined method of data-analysis. The more we allow our research 'subjects' to participate in defining what is to count as data, the more we have to turn to flexible ways of categorising and sorting the often unexpected things we are told and observe. As we saw in chapter 7, researchers such as Kitzinger (1994) describe the people who participated in their focus group studies as 'co-researchers'. In the delicate task of getting inside people's experience, these 'co-researchers' can take the lead, with the researchers following. And this includes the analysis of data. Indeed, it is common for researchers working with community groups to test the validity of their own analysis by taking it back to the community for comment and verification. They may even go back repeatedly, with the subjects' comment on the analysis in itself providing further data (Mays & Pope 1995b). Cynics may wonder who takes ultimate responsibility for this recursive process — or even who draws the research salary. On the other hand, the process of involving the community intimately in the research process can in itself constitute an intervention resulting in community action to improve its own health — hence the term 'action research'.

The issue of researcher bias takes on a new dimension in such studies. Some researchers commit themselves not to representing a balanced public health view of an issue but to giving a deeply engaged account of the lives of people — often people living in misery, the 'underdogs', the people all too often, and too conveniently, overlooked in other methods. Chapter 6 discussed the account of mothering among users of crack cocaine (Kearney et al. 1994). The aim of the study was to conduct the research from a feminist perspective, recognising the needs that women themselves identify, with the goal of women's 'personal and political empowerment' (p. 352). Their conclusion called for increased access to 'survival-level resources' and for support in keeping the family intact while the women tried to come to grips with the problems in their lives. This study is certainly innovative in the strength of its commitment to representing the women's views, but it was not classified as truly innovative because there did not appear to be any ongoing relationship with the women, the researchers themselves conducted the analysis (although they did take some aspects of the analysis back to the women for comment), and they called for policy change rather than engaging in community action. When we step into the territory of the innovators, this distancing between researcher and participants in the analysis can be forfeited, and so can the appeal for policy change rather than direct action.

Despite the interest with which we view the efforts of these innovators, it is not true to say that they go on their innovative way without any methodological guidance. Ethnographic methods developed out of the field work of anthropologists studying unfamiliar communities (see Hammersley & Atkinson 1983). A number of the studies described below make explicit use of ethnographic methods; others draw on a range of methods, often including participant observation, a quintessentially ethnographic tool. A brief discussion of ethnographic method, therefore, provides a good methodological starting point for reviewing innovative qualitative studies.

Ethnography is the classic method for studying a social or cultural niche about which we know very little. Researchers commit themselves to seeing things from the perspective of the people involved. The methods used are an eclectic combination, including interviews, observation, and documentary analysis (Fielding 1993). The method is reflexive — that is, researchers are part of the social setting, and data are analysed by switching between involved participation and detached analysis.

Steps for ethnographic fieldwork
- Define a role (researcher, participant, or other) that balances participation with detached observation, without deception.
- Negotiate entry to the field.
- Record the action, usually in field notes.
- Analyse the data, searching for patterns and themes.
- Check on the validity of data and analysis in a self-critical way.
- Write the story (often in the first person).

Some examples

The first study uses an ethnographic approach in a new and challenging way. In the personal interviews they conducted, the researchers showed an unusual degree of involvement with a group of vulnerable research participants: parents with 'learning difficulties' (Booth & Booth 1994). Twenty unstructured interviews were conducted to obtain a biographical account of their experiences as parents. Six couples and a single mother were selected for further study. The researchers noted that the life-story approach they chose to use cannot be a 'hit and run' affair; it is time-consuming and intensive, but it is unusual in the public health literature to find researchers who take the task as seriously as this team did. The researchers set out to gain the trust of their 'informants', but they also felt it important to establish as much rapport as possible. The task required 126 interviews, fifteen social calls, 121 telephone calls, and twenty-two trips and outings — but it was worthwhile:

> we treated rapport as a two-way process of communication involving both information gathering and giving. We were happy to give people our home address and telephone number, and to let them know we would be pleased to hear from them if ever they wanted to contact us (and many did) . . . Both [trust and rapport] may have a fundamental bearing on what and how much people are prepared to disclose. Informants may have many things they would ordinarily hide from a stranger and a myriad reasons for garnishing the truth. One mother, for example, only began to talk about her first child, who had been taken away at birth, after eight interviews. Rather than being an indulgence, trust and rapport may have a crucial influence on the quality of the data obtained (Booth & Booth 1994: 417–18).

The researchers had to live up to this commitment, dealing with the problem of being seen as potential benefactors and, finally, negotiating to withdraw from the close personal relationships built up in the course of doing the research only at a pace set by their informants.

The ground rules for the first of what they call 'meetings' rather than 'interviews' were these:

- Take your cue from the informant and be prepared to adapt according to their emotional needs and responses.
- Generally speaking, just listening is the best approach.
- Do not go in with a predetermined set of questions to ask or topics to discuss.
- Allow the informant to dictate what and how much is talked about.
- Do not feel pressured to record; you can always return to points again later.
- Any data collected at the first meeting should be regarded as a bonus (p. 418).

With a longer term commitment to ongoing contact with informants, the emphasis did not need to fall as heavily on tape recording of interviews; rather, researchers could concentrate on listening and exploit the extra freedom of being able to move around or cope with background noise.

How is the validity of the data assured in a study such as this? The researchers described it as follows:

> Making comparisons between families was perhaps the best technique for validating the experiential data: as one account confirms another, *stories accrete and regularities emerge* so it becomes less likely that individual narratives are the product of one person's fancy and more likely that they show structural features in the lives of the subjects.
>
> Over and above these technical checks on the data, however, there remains the feeling human observer. Ultimately, in this type of research, the validity of the data is the stuff of the relationship between the interviewer and the informant. Someone who phones the researcher to ask when they are going to see each other again is unlikely to be an evasive respondent (p. 421, emphasis added).

The researchers describe their methods as fairly standard, but what is new is that 'people with learning difficulties' are seldom seen as capable informants: 'our study points the way to a new ethnography which accords them the status of actors in the drama of their own lives and gives them a voice in the making of their own history' (p. 423).

While this study used different forms of contact to ensure trust and rapport, these can in themselves provide additional sources of data, as in the study by Borkan and co-workers (1995), a study of patients' experiences of low-back pain. They conducted focus groups and individual interviews, selecting participants from three kibbutzim in Israel through purposeful sampling — that is, selecting people who are knowledgeable about the topic and willing to be interviewed. At the same time, the researchers participated in the activities of the kibbutzim, taking part in agricultural labour, work drafts, and dining-hall duty, all the while discussing how the community saw low-back pain and its relationship to work. A similar study was conducted in three communities in South Wales about community views on the prevention of cardiac disease (Davison et al. 1992). This study used interviews, observation and participation in local activities, informal contact with residents, and many unstructured conversations, which showed that knowledge of behavioural risk was not reflected in people's personal lifestyle.

Both these studies aimed to elucidate the community culture with respect to illness, but in studies with a high degree of community participation, the community itself is likely to undergo change as participants and researchers exchange insights. A study in Kinshasa, Zaire, conducted what the researchers called 'intervention ethnography'. While discussing AIDS with communities, they provided information on prevention and observed people's responses (Schoepf 1993). They note that 'dialogue with informants produced rich texts about resistance to change' (p. 1403), and this was used to devise ways of addressing constraints, such as the cultural expectations of sexual partners. Among the research approaches they used were role plays, case studies, and simulation games. With a group of church women, the role of the cajoling wife was played by a young sex worker, but they later found out that the grandmother who played the resistant husband had also been a sex worker. Thus they brought skills to their role-playing of which the researchers were initially unaware, but which formed an important part of the action research:

> Grounded in group dynamics, action-research in the original meaning of the term uses experiential, or process training to stimulate personal and social change. It begins with the principle that people already know a great deal about their own situations. It builds upon this knowledge, using processes of social interaction to develop a 'critical consciousness' about human behavior and the causes of social phenomena (p. 1403).

A paper by Seeley and others (1992) offers a note of caution about community participation in the sensitive area of HIV/AIDS research in rural Uganda. From community participation, a research program gains local knowledge and access to people who provide an entrée to the community and help resolve political issues as they occur. However, these programs often remain foreign, externally imposed, and there is the risk that the research will draw people away from important community tasks and roles. The ideal of full participation in a research agenda set by the community is hard to reach. And yet, a study of workers' health using participatory methods in Mexico City argues that collective consciousness-raising and change are direct results of methodologies that include collective discussion with workers about the measures required to improve working conditions and health (Laurell et al. 1992).

In many studies, of course, the idea that the community should take action is inappropriate. An example here is a study that looks at the downside of the public health emphasis on risk (Handwerker 1994). The problem that sparked off the study was a case in San Diego, California, in which a poor woman was arrested, gaoled, and charged with medical neglect of the foetus she was carrying. She had disregarded medical advice and engaged in what was seen as 'high-risk' behaviour. A court's ability to charge women with prenatal child-abuse has significant implications for poor pregnant women seeking antenatal care. Working from data collected by participant observation, informal conversations, open-ended interviews, and information from local newspapers, the researcher defined the different meanings assigned to 'risky' behaviour. While practitioners are concerned with apparently objective scientific fact, for the women as risk-takers, the problem is one of making sense of ambiguous epidemiological evidence in the context of the constraints of their everyday lives. Here it is the law that has to change.

Many ethnographic studies use multiple methods. A study conducted in the Bagamoya District, Tanzania, aimed to promote the use of insecticide-impregnated mosquito nets (Winch et al. 1994). They supplemented focus groups and key informant interviews with a range of inventive methods for gauging local views on seasons, seasonal variations in mosquito populations, and incidence of fever. Their aim was to develop culturally appropriate ways of emphasising the need for bed nets. A more complex study using multiple methods involves the abuse of high-dose hormonal drugs as a covert abortifacient in Cusco, Peru (Bonnema & Dalebout 1992). This practice is banned in Western countries because of the risk of birth defects. In order to uncover this use of the drugs, the Spanish-speaking researchers carried out an inventory of the availability of these drugs in Cusco, as well as conducting discussions with women and pharmacists. Presenting themselves as medical students conducting a study of the use of medicines in gynaecology and obstetrics, they were able to gain access to outpatient clinics, where they observed 112 consultations by doctors and fifty-three by midwives. These practitioners and others were interviewed. They then hired a woman from Cusco to pose as a fake patient and buy the drug without prescription from pharmacies. They showed serious abuses of the drugs.

If ethnographic methods are useful for studying people who are usually not seen as capable of being good informants, they should also be useful in studying groups who may be resistant to giving information on their 'socially undesirable behaviour'. A study of needle-sharing in the Netherlands formed part of a study of the drug-taking rituals of heroin 'addicts' (Grund et al. 1991). There were no formal interviews; the study used 'street ethnography' as well as 'intense participant observation' involving a field worker described as 'a respected ex-addict'. The risk of being caught in periodic drug raids appears to have been compensated for by access to detailed information on drug-using rituals. The observation of illicit routines is clearly a tricky issue. The researchers had to be acceptable to the group, participating in its activities, but we are not told what this involved. Moore (1993) conducted a similar study with young, recreational illicit drug-users in Perth. He describes himself as 'moving with' the group, but again does not provide further detail on the extent of participation.

One can safely assume that it is the risk involved in participation in some settings that leads researchers to turn instead to non-participant observation. And, indeed, if non-participant observation is sufficient, why take the risk of participating? An intriguing study from Managua (Gorter et al. 1993) involved collecting condoms from motel rooms after the occupants had left and inspecting them to see if they contained semen. The condoms had been provided to clients at check-in. For seven hours on each of five days, researchers also observed the number of couples entering and the time spent in each room in five motels. Seamark and Gaughwin (1994) examined fifty-eight syringes found in prisons in Adelaide. Prison officers confiscated the syringes during routine searches and delivered them to the authors. Examination of the syringes indicated multiple use. Less risky was the observation of seating patterns on the Washington Metropolitan Rail System, which showed that children seemed to favour the safer rear-facing seats (Trinkoff 1985). An observation study of salt-use at dining tables by Mittelmark and Sternberg (1985) was followed by a questionnaire, which showed that people accurately reported their use of salt.

Observation is also a common method of study in clinical settings. A classic example is the study of Bloor (1976), in which he observed ear, nose, and throat surgeons to see how they made their decisions on when to operate. Understanding the decision-making process contributed to understanding geographical variation in surgery rates (Mays & Pope 1995a). It is common in studies of this kind for the researchers to supplement their observations with tape-recordings of clinical consultations.

A problem here is that it may be more difficult to persuade medical colleagues to allow this intrusion into their realm of power than it is to persuade a local community group. Researchers who have managed this include Silverman (1987), who describes a series of such studies, and Mishler (1984), who concentrated on close analysis of speech in such encounters. Danziger (1979) describes the joys of 'doctor-watching' in medical settings. Heath (1986) pushes this analysis to its limits by showing how video recordings of consultations can be transcribed to capture gestures, body movement, and eye contact. Let the enthusiast beware: a few seconds of conversation give a page of transcription.

Embedded in conversations recorded during consultations can be found patient narratives — the stories people tell about their experience of illness. Waitzkin and Britt (1993), for example, used narrative methods to analyse patient–doctor discourses about so-called 'self-destructive behavior' (smoking, substance-use, and sexual practices). For Viney and Bousfield (1991), collecting and analysing narrative accounts of illness is the response of researchers who feel that the 'lists of numbers and stuff' simply are 'not me'. People use language to interpret their own experience for themselves and for others, to express feelings, and to maintain relationships. In other words, language constructs meanings, and the texts of narrative accounts are therefore well worth analysing. The Viney and Bousfield paper gives a detailed description of methods of analysing narratives from AIDS-affected people.

Hassin (1994) focused her analysis on the account of one intravenous drug-user (from a large ethnographic study) who used her HIV-positive diagnosis to redefine her social identity in a positive way. She described herself as looking forward to her future as a mother: 'You know that's why I'm kinda glad I went through some of the things I went through because now I want to be my daughter's friend. I . . . want her to be able to come to me when there is something wrong' (p. 395). Similarly, Riessman (1990) shows the way in which a self is constituted through narrative by analysing an account of divorce as experienced by one working-class man with advanced multiple sclerosis.

Marshall and O'Keefe (1995) turned the self-narrative method on its head by asking medical students to write their own narrative accounts after hearing the account of a patient with AIDS, and then they analysed the medical narratives. In Cape Town, South Africa, Lerer and colleagues (1995) produced a telling account of infant deaths by analysing the accounts taken down by police when poor Black families came to register these deaths. Connell and others (1991) showed, through an analysis of life histories, how being working class impacts on gay men and AIDS prevention.

We are now in methodological territory that is sociological rather than anthropological. Sociologists have found the use of life histories useful in the analysis of chronic disease. A series of papers on qualitative research on chronic illness, published in *Social Science and Medicine*, provides an excellent overview of this field. Included in the 1990 issue are an overview of method and conceptual development by Conrad, a study of multiple sclerosis by Robinson, and a study of long-stay hospital and nursing-home care by Clark and Bowling.

Gerhardt's study (1990) of the experience of end-stage renal disease is a particularly useful example for further discussion because of the care with which she discusses conceptual details. She argues that medical sociologists have all too often assumed, on the basis of studies done in other contexts, that chronic illness is a form of social deviance, characterised by stigmatisation and exclusion. Rather she sees the way in which patients with chronic disease lead their lives as much less marked by stigma and social exclusion than has been allowed by compassionate sociologists. She draws on the sociological notion of a patient 'career' — a trajectory of events in the course of the illness over time — with patients using adaptive strategies to 'normalise' or cope with the threat to life and livelihood. In the light of improved medical care, these social strategies allow patients and their families to maintain a state of normal or near-normal social participation.

Gerhardt's focus is on married patients with end-stage renal disease, and she documents changes over the course of about five years in treatment, identity-management, socio-economic normalisation, and the role of the family in coping with change. With sixty-seven patients in the interview study, 234 tape-recorded interviews were conducted with patients and spouses. For most she had eight hours or more of biographical information on the chronological course of their lives. Hospital data over twelve years were also available.

Gerhardt describes her method of analysis in detail. The problem was to develop a general account of different experiences. She did not want to break the data up by coding and sorting into categories because this would break the 'time-flow of the life stories'. Instead she analysed entire cases, examining them for the dynamics involved. She drew on what has been termed 'grand theory' — in this case, Max Weber's notion of the ideal type, developed in response to understanding historical material, but never before used in empirical research. An ideal type, briefly, is a 'synthesis of a great many diffuse, discrete, more or less present and occasionally absent concrete individual phenomena, which are arranged according to . . . one-sidedly emphasized viewpoints into a unified analytical construct' (p. 1214). Following this device, the focus of analysis was to define those career patterns associated with 'optimal survival outcome'. At issue here was the family's occupational rehabilitation (changes to maintain family income), treatment options (transplantation versus continuing dialysis) and marital status (whether the marriage survives).

One further paper in the series is worth noting for its description of an unusual qualitative method that Armstrong (1990) describes as follows: '[a] method which does not observe or listen to the patient for the truth he or she might reveal, but instead explores the relationship between the words the patient utters and the techniques used to elicit those words' (p. 1225). Armstrong calls this the 'genealogical method' after the work of the theorist Michel Foucault. It involves analysing the social conditions under which it became possible to recognise 'chronic disease' and the institutional frameworks within which the category was, and is, used. He argues that chronic illness was uncovered by the use of morbidity surveys. The conditions for its existence are intimately linked to surveys that asked people 'Are you ill?' or 'In the last two weeks, did you have to cut down on any of the things you usually do because of illness or injury?'. The next step then is to link the methodology of the health questionnaire to techniques of production — in this case the development of prevention and screening techniques. In Armstrong's formulation, method does not illuminate; it fabricates. And this process of fabrication is, in itself, worth studying.

Advantages and disadvantages

The advantage of being innovative is that there are no constraints placed on what is seen as possible, and the studies outlined above bear witness to the inventiveness of the mind of the public health researcher. With researchers prepared to depart from the path of the tested and true, there are few public health problems for which we cannot find an appropriate method of study. But researchers will need staying power for the intensive longitudinal studies.

Many of the studies described above are driven by what might be called a political commitment: to show the pain of the ill and the injustice experienced by the oppressed. But what is there to divide the researcher from the political activist? It is probably worth noting here that much public health research is driven by commitment and a need to change things for the better. The only difference is that this is seldom acknowledged in classical study designs. Many public health researchers take an objective stance, which apparently precludes them from implementing their findings; some even fail to spell out what the policy implications of their research are at all. Perhaps these differences can be resolved by agreeing that public health research is, indeed, a political act — we want to bring about change — but that this should be achieved in a methodologically respectable manner.

This, of course, does not let the qualitative innovator off the hook. The answer to the problems of innovative research is the same as it is for every other method: methodological rigour in the conduct of our research. Whatever the method of sample selection, researchers need to recognise the limitations that their method imposes on the results. The issue of validity of data is addressed in terms of the sensitivity of the relationship between researcher and researched-upon, an unusual concept for many public health researchers. The reliability of the analysis depends upon its acceptance by the study participants, on the degree to which it brings about positive change in the study community, or even on the extent to which the analysis is accepted by public health peers. There are no secure rules to follow here, but that does not mean that issues of rigour do not remain at the forefront of the research task.

One of the differences between these studies and the more traditional qualitative studies is that innovative researchers tend to resist the 'shattering' of data through processes of coding and categorising. Instead the stress falls on the integrity of the story, analysed by the use of conceptual categories. To some extent, according to Conrad (1990), understanding the patient's life-world is sacrificed to make sociological and conceptual sense of the account. On the other hand, he sees the issue of generalisability in terms of the generalisability of the concepts used in the analysis. So, for example, conceptual notions like the disavowal of 'deviance' or 'stigma' to describe people's experience may be applicable across a range of chronic illnesses in other samples, settings, or situations.

> **Advantages of qualitative innovations**
> - They offer freedom from methodological blinkering.
> - A research approach can be matched to a wide range of research problems.
>
> **Disadvantages of qualitative innovations**
> - There is a lack of tried and tested methodological guides.
> - It is sometimes difficult to determine when research becomes activism.
> - Generalisability can be uncertain.

Issues of ethics

It is not clear why some researchers cheat and deceive in the conduct of their research. At first sight, working with innovative qualitative methods seems to offer extraordinary opportunity to practise methodological fraud. However, we should remember that there is not a method that effectively guards against this problem in *any* methodological area. Indeed, it is perhaps easier to invent phantom laboratory rabbits than phantom communities, who can speak up and comment on their own participation.

One of the perennial problems with participant observation is the question of covert observation — that is, when the people being observed are unaware that it is happening. There is only one study among the examples discussed in this chapter that acknowledges deception — the case in which a fake patient approached pharmacies for a drug (Bonnema & Dalebout 1992) — but this was, perhaps, in a good cause. This is certainly an issue that requires further discussion for its ethical implications.

Perhaps the most serious ethical consideration involves the degree of involvement between researcher and community. Some of the studies mentioned, including the study of parents with learning difficulties (Booth & Booth 1994), give an excellent account of the degree to which the researchers carefully considered their obligations to their research participants. While this is clearly a serious issue for the innovative public health researcher, we should balance this concern with the recognition that it is common practice for researchers doing laboratory studies to take specimens of blood or body tissue from research subjects and then never inform them of the results of the study. With these qualitative methods, at least some of the participants stand to gain an increased understanding of their own experience, and if they do not like what is happening during the research process, they can vote with their feet.

Recommended reading

Duffy, M. & Hedin, B. 1988, 'New Directions for Nursing Research', in N. Woods & M. Catanzaro (eds), *Nursing Research: Theory and Practice*, C.V. Mosby, St Louis, Mo.
   A volume worth reading for the nursing approach to innovative research.
Fielding, N. 1993, 'Ethnography', in N. Gilbert (ed.), *Researching Social Life*, Sage, London.
Hammersley, M. & Atkinson, P. 1983, *Ethnography: Principles in Practice*, Tavistock, London.
   A well-used text.
Kitzinger, J. 1994, 'The Methodology of Focus Groups: The Importance of Interaction between Research Participants', *Sociology of Health and Illness*, vol. 16, no. 1, pp. 103–21.
   An excellent overview and critique.
Mays, N. & Pope, C. 1995a, 'Observational Methods in Health Care Settings', *British Medical Journal*, vol. 311, 15 July, pp. 182–4.
—— 1995b, 'Rigour and Qualitative Research', *British Medical Journal*, vol. 311, 8 July, pp. 109–12.
   Part of an excellent set of overview articles published over successive weeks.
Mies, M. 1983, 'Towards a Methodology for Feminist Research', in G. Bowles & R. Klein (eds), *Theories of Women's Studies*, Routledge & Kegan Paul, London.

CHAPTER 12

Innovations from Cultural and Social Studies

Whoever said 'medicine is a social science' had only half the story, but a very good idea nevertheless. This is because each clinical science is not one thing, but is simultaneously several things. Clinical practitioners are engaged in both a science and an art; they must balance an academic understanding of universal physical processes with the clinical realities of the unique case before them. And in coming to an understanding of that single case, the clinician does well to remember that the person under examination is a social and cultural being, whose life and behaviour cannot be properly understood using methods designed to understand the atom, the Krebs cycle, or the processes of inflammation and repair.

Because much of what we need to understand about health and illness is social, a significant proportion of what passes for public health is really social science rather than medical science. And this is as it should be, if for no other reason than that it matches our most relevant methods with our most wily and slippery questions. The ambiguity inherent in the pursuit of public health answers has led, unfortunately, to a certain stubborn attachment to the methods of physical science. This has encouraged an equally regrettable and narrow set of methodological attitudes. Let us apply the randomised control trial in whatever home will have it. Let a survey go out into the world and measure whatever will be measured. Let us talk to whoever will tell us things. And in all these matters, let us count what counts as valuable data to our colleagues in medical science. But there *are* other ways to study public health.

In the preceeding chapters, we have identified and described some of the more common examples, images, and techniques associated with conventional social science approaches to public health, particularly qualitative methods. It is commonly thought that public health equals surveys, randomised control trials, and quantitative data-analysis, and social science's contribution has commonly been associated with some of these approaches and with the qualitative methodologies. But in this final chapter, we will demonstrate that social and cultural studies have more to offer the public health researcher than simply qualitative methods. The humanities and social sciences have further ways of viewing and analysing data and data sources — ways that provide the behavioural and clinical sciences with an opportunity to expand their understanding of the concept of 'good science'.

Good science and quality public health research

Good science in public health tends to be identified with the 'hypothetico-deductive' model of research. First, a person, or persons, read up on the subject (this is the literature review). After this, the researchers get an idea or two that they would like to test (the theoretical framework or hypotheses). So they go out into the world (with a method or two), test their ideas (get some results), and see if they were right in the first place (the discussion).

Of course, this model of good science is based on three well-known philosophical positions: empiricism (the idea that you should 'go' somewhere to get answers), positivism (the idea that, when you get there, you ought to measure something), and rationalism (the idea that a major purpose of the desire to measure is to ascertain a cause-and-effect relation). This view of science worked wonderfully for topics and issues for which universal principles might be discerned. It worked well for chemistry and physics, for example. But it did not, and does not, work well for other sciences.

Another model of good science was developed for trickier scientific problems: the 'descriptive-inductive' model. In this model, researchers also read as much as they could, to familiarise themselves with an issue (literature review). But all that reading is then teamed up with some substantial observations, from which hypotheses or conclusions might later be drawn (descriptive observations). This particular approach was based on three slightly different philosophies: empiricism (once again, reaffirming the need to go somewhere — in this case, into 'habitats'), phenomenology (so as to gain an understanding of the organism's point of view), and interactionism (to identify and describe the factors in the subjects' environment, which might account for why they behave the way they do). This view of science worked beautifully with topics and issues for which the context was crucial to any understanding. It worked well for environmental science, marine biology, and anthropology, for example. In the social sciences, this particular approach goes by the label 'qualitative' research.

The clinical, behavioural, and social sciences have employed these two models of science with varying success for some time now. Medicine has preferred the 'hypothetico-deductive' model more than the social sciences, and has not always appreciated the fact that what is now called the 'qualitative' approach has, in fact, been used by the natural sciences for a longer time. These two models or approaches to science, however, do not exhaust the paradigms that might be used to extend a researcher's enquiries.

The humanities — that other collection of 'sciences' developed during the European Enlightenment in the sixteenth and seventeenth centuries (Toulmin 1990) — offer some useful lessons for the public health researcher. Their concern with language, story, art, or music, as well as with questions of sense and sensibility within these forms of representation, have provided us with yet another way of understanding the human creature at work and play. These 'deconstructive' models, like their qualitative cousins, highlight styles of scientific analysis already embedded and existing in clinical thought and practice.

Derived from psychoanalysis and literary theory, deconstructive models draw on the central idea that behaviour and meanings can frequently be hidden — indeed, even one's own meaning can be hidden from oneself. People do not always have a meaning or reason for what they do, whether the behaviour be simple, such as twiddling one's fingers, or far more complex, such as getting married. In these cases, the curious must approach the hazardous interpretive domains of history, artwork, or poetry to uncover, in whatever shadowy and imperfect way, the subterranean, cultural influences on emotion and motive.

The meaning *behind* the story or behaviour must be revealed, and there are a number of strategies that one can employ to do this. People in every science, including medicine, intuitively know and use these strategies in their own ways. Just as one might use symptoms and signs to probe beneath surface appearances and make a clinical assessment, one can gently probe and identify ideas and language as signifiers of underlying messages and desires. One can also manipulate these structures through the deliberate and evocative employment of particular ideas and language. While this insight is well understood by film and television producers, as well as musicians and advertising executives, it is not an insight explicitly recognised, understood, or debated by public health researchers.

The insights and skills involved in this style of work have belonged mainly to those from philosophy, history, and literary studies, and more recently from areas with new names: cultural studies, women's studies, postmodern social theory, and media studies. There has been much criticism and debate about the use and validity of analysing symbolic representations such as personal styles or cultural products, but this is not the place to assess these matters. It is sufficient to point out that each of the above scientific models has proved valuable to its peddlers. Let us not forget, for example, that while the hypothetico-deductive model of science gave us the automobile, it was insights from literary and then media studies that sold them to us in prodigious numbers. Both scientific models have produced compelling 'results'.

What the public health researcher might gain from this quick overview of the various models of good science is that these models do not so much compete as represent three poorly recognised sides of a single model of good science — a model that we all use in practice. In our failure to recognise that we do, in fact, use all three models of science, we have given more 'press' to just one approach: the hypothetico-deductive model. In so doing, we have largely overlooked, downplayed, or misunderstood the role that other aspects of our science have played in the task of discovery.

If we were now to give those aspects of good science the recognition that they deserve, how could public health researchers draw on these approaches? In the remainder of this chapter, we will re-examine the deconstructive arts and identify the key features that have relevance to public health research. These can be summarised as follows:

1 Research does not have to involve live people; it can be unobtrusive. Few scholars in literary theory or philosophy interview or survey people. Instead they make use of examining what they call the 'text' — that is, the story as revealed in the printed word.

2 Because culture is not considered to be 'out there' but everywhere, everything is potential data. Film, television, physical objects, architectural design, facial expressions, novels, personal diaries, and so on.
3 The key way to analyse this material is not necessarily through some positivistic tradition of content-analysis, but rather through the equally complex world of semiotics — the 'science' or 'art' of interpreting.

We will now review some examples of existing public health research that have made pioneering inroads into this new area. We will first examine the public health researcher's interest in text, and then discuss a wider interest in other examples of popular culture and their perceived relevance to public health. Finally, we will review some introductory, practical principles for semiotic analysis in public health research.

Unobtrusive research in public health

When we discussed secondary analysis in chapter 9, we remarked in passing that this particular methodology included the analysis of printed materials other than numerical data, especially newspapers and professional literature. We will take some time now to examine some of this material in closer detail.

Carey and others (1994) examined how competing interest groups framed their arguments in the debate over pool fencing in New South Wales. In a study that has powerful and practical implications for future health advocacy and policy, Carey and his colleagues show how those who opposed fencing employed the same non-interventionist arguments and philosophy that the government of the day expressed with regard to other social issues. The pro-fencing groups' refusal to compromise on the issue of retrospective fencing is shown to have been an important factor in galvanising opposition to them. The debate is examined and traced in fine detail through the newspapers and parliamentary records of the day. The shifting positions can be closely linked to the nature, tenor, and amount of argument and support from each of the warring factions.

Chapman and company (1995) examined the occurrence of insidious, incidental advertising for smoking in popular magazines after the ban on tobacco advertising in January 1991. They examined twenty Australian magazines for young people and for those from lower socio-economic groups. They sampled for three periods: 1990 (before the ban), and 1991 and 1993 (after the ban). Initially, over the period 1990–91, there was a 75 per cent increase in the rate of photographs depicting smoking, and then between 1991 and 1993, there was a 36 per cent reduction. Some magazines showed no photographs of people smoking at all, and this highlights the possibility that others in the magazine business will also improve.

Lupton (1995) analysed a year's worth of front-page medical and health stories in the *Sydney Morning Herald* to gauge their nature and slant. In this case study of Sydney's best-selling broadsheet, Lupton argued that the paper privileged the medical voice (the male voice in that context); gave less space to advocacy, activist, and community groups; and tended to individualise illness rather than link it to broader socio-economic or political contexts. It seems that the 'new' public health is not news to the *Sydney Morning Herald*.

Penetrating beyond the front-page story, Lupton and Chapman (1995) examined a brace of newspaper stories provided by the newspaper-clipping service of the Australian National Heart Foundation. They found contradictory and confusing messages about coronary health. At times, news stories supported public health messages, but at other times they were critical, even cynical, about them. This trend was reflected in popular attitudes measured by Lupton and Chapman in their focus group research. Other studies in which researchers have raked through newspapers for health message content include examinations of press coverage of alcohol and breast cancer (Houn et al. 1995); of publications on smoking (Chapman 1989) and smokers' rights (Cardador et al. 1995); and of the coverage of AIDS in the French press (Herzlich & Pierret, 1989).

Some public health researchers have preferred to analyse literature closer to home: their own professional literature. Webb and others (1990) conducted a critical review of the public education material produced by Australian cancer organisations. They found that there was a lack of agreement about risk groups, prevention, timing of screening, and even what action is recommended if a sign or symptom is discovered.

Skolbekken (1995) examined the frequency of the term 'risk' in the medical literature and found that the use of this term can literally be described as epidemic. This increased use of the term cannot be accounted for by changes in terminology alone. Our beliefs about the nature and extent of personal control over disease and misfortune have shifted markedly. Skolbekken examines the historical and cultural factors underlying that shift.

Kleinman and Cohen (1991) examined the portrayal of mental illness in advertisements appearing in the *American Journal of Psychiatry*. They found a preponderance of stereotypical and decontextualised images, as well as distorted ideas about treatment and treatment options. These representations contribute to greater, rather than less, ignorance in general social relations and attitudes towards mental illness.

Finally, Van Trigt and many others (1995) compared the medical literature with newspapers in their coverage of medicines. They found that medical journals gave more press to negative consequences of medicines than did newspapers. The more positive newspaper portrayal of these drugs might contribute to the public's ignorance or apathy about prescribed and over-the-counter drugs and their potential ill effects.

So, what observations can we make about these unusual examples of secondary analysis? First, we must recognise the positive and practical contribution of much of this material. Secondary analysis of textual material makes obvious contributions to health-care evaluation (as did the study of the health-promotional material produced by cancer organisations, for instance); to health policy development (the 'discourse'-analysis of pool fencing advocates and their opponents, for example); to health sociology (as demonstrated by the cultural analysis of the proliferation of 'risk' — one of public health's most cherished concepts); and to health and medical education (as did the review of advertising images in psychiatric journals).

Second, most of these analyses are eclectic (but not unsystematic) in their methodological styles. Unlike other examples of public health methodology, the secondary analysis of textual material shows an admirable and pioneering respect for approaches other than the hypothetico-deductive approach. There are, of course, also standard content-analysis approaches, in which positivist researchers search for their preconceived and pre-theorised categories, measuring columns of newsprint here and number of words there. But other researchers seek to identify themes that emerge from the texts as a function of the text's own editorial slant, bias, or organisational policy. And in tracing, describing, and theorising about those influences, a deconstructive approach emerges that is both provocative and original, and that shapes future research with a greater measurement orientation.

Third, the emphasis on penetrating beneath the text's surface has encouraged and privileged the public health tradition of social criticism. Ironically, the hypothetico-deductive approaches have led to a concern with describing results, while the descriptive and deconstructive approaches, demonstrated by the above examples, have led to critiques of people's living conditions. This is an academic approach that was characteristic of the 'old' public health — which was critical of the sanitation, work, and housing deficits of poor communities — but is seldom seen in the discussion of results in the latest randomised control trials.

But the literature that people read — and consequently the ideas that surround modern peoples — leads us once again to the need to resurrect the critical tradition that focuses on environments and living conditions. This brings us to our final observation about these data sources and their corresponding methods of analysis.

The textual analysis of literature recognises that much Western health education and promotion occurs through, and is mediated by, printed materials in both popular and professional forums. A much-needed critical examination of this modern nexus has only just begun, and the few studies mentioned here as illustrations demonstrate that there is much to be gained from such an examination. The primary insight to be gained from adapting this aspect of humanities scholarship to public health is that much of the 'public' at the centre of what we call 'public health' is a reading public. The full implication of this insight for public health research is yet to be realised.

Cultural studies and public health

Of course, the printed word includes more than just newspapers or professional literature. Almost any text can be explored for its public health insights. Koutroulis's study (1990) of gynaecological textbooks and their portrayal of women is ample evidence of that. Nevertheless, the extent of cultural production and influence is merely touched upon by examinations of the printed word. For even the printed word is only one step up from the abstraction of social life represented in numerical data sets. There comes a time when it is both useful and necessary to look physically at the humanity at the centre of our attentions.

Campbell and others (1995) and Irish and Hall (1995) are just two examples of public health researchers who have decided to look directly at human interactions — in these cases, interactions in medical consultations. These researchers have videotaped consultations to examine patterns of consultation and their effects on patients. Their observations, and their subsequent interpretations, have the added advantage of being very reliable in that these data are clearly amenable to careful inter-rater checks.

Conducted along similarly preconceived lines are Story and Faulkner's content-analysis study of eating behaviour and food messages on prime-time television (1990); Hazan and others' study of the portrayal of tobacco-use in sixty-two of the top-grossing United States films from 1960 to 1990 (1994); Reid's simple observations of nurses' interactions with mothers and children in Papua New Guinean maternal and child clinics (1984); and finally, Threlfall's very clever study (1992), which photographed people waiting at a kerb to cross at lights in order to determine whether their clothing arrangements reflected the public 'slip, slop, slap' anti-cancer campaign in Australia.

Other studies that assume that the non-verbal culture all around us is worth studying include the numerous computer modelling projects that employ artificial-intelligence software to model, for example, disease outbreak information; or alternatively, the public health researchers who study material culture, such as those who examine the physical consequences of cyclone damage (Finau et al. 1986); or those who examine automobile crash sites (Ryan et al. 1992) or car designs and their health consequences (Society of Automotive Engineers 1996).

All these studies examined actual behaviours as these appeared on video, in still photos, in film, or in real life. None involved interviews or administered surveys, but most of them began with some idea or category of behaviour that they wished to detect, measure, and report on. Despite the use of largely positivist, preconceived designs, they represent an important departure from conventional public health research and an equally important move towards cultural studies. Nevertheless, if the designs were more qualitative or deconstructivist, more could be asked of this research.

As examples, let us re-examine the previously mentioned studies. In Story and Faulkner's (1990) content-analysis of food messages and scenes on prime-time television, all items are treated as if they were of equal interest to viewers. Advertisements have the same influential weight as sit-coms. There is little attempt to distinguish between television characters or plots. Clearly some characters depend on viewers identifying with them, and producers attempt to mirror their viewers' habits rather than send new messages. This is the opposite of the intentions of many advertisements. There is no attempt to use context to assess the message being sent. And even though Story and Faulkner accept that most food incidents on television are 'trivial and incidental', such incidents are not distinguished from those that are not. Focusing less on trivial items and providing a more descriptive analysis of main meal episodes may have provided different results.

Hazan and colleagues (1994) observed their smoking characters closely and noted that ashtrays were slowly disappearing in smoking scenes. So what? More relevant questions to focus on might have been: How were the non-smoking characters portrayed? What new objects were replacing the ashtray? What messages did these alternative symbols and people send? In concentrating too firmly on the presence of images in which the researchers were interested, they may have neglected other important dimensions that a casual viewer could regard as important.

Reid (1984) made interesting observations of mothers' and children's behaviour in maternal and child-care clinics in Papua New Guinea, but she did so as a White anthropologist. How much of what she observed was a function of a continuing Melanesian performance before an ongoing White surveillance — a colonising surveillance that many Papuans have grown used to in the health area?

And finally, Threlfall (1992) conducts a fascinating content-analysis of photographs of people standing on kerbs waiting to cross the road. He wants to know how successful the public health, anti-skin-cancer campaign to 'cover up' has been with ordinary people. He notes that the message to cover up appears to be understood, but in very limited ways. His analysis does not take into account the influence of competing 'campaigns', such as fashion industry campaigns and the gendered clothing messages that appear daily in magazines and on television. The cultural context of people's dress sense is not examined alongside his analysis of photos of people on the kerb. And yet, without this other dimension, without that context, we have results that are very limited in their ability to speak to us about how popular culture influences health. But it does not have to be this way.

The public health researchers in the previous examples see obvious merit in researching the same objects of study as those targeted by cultural studies, but they focus specifically on meanings of health as opposed to the host of other topics that might interest others in the humanities. But the deconstructive style of data-analysis — which is present in some examples of secondary analysis of newspapers from a public health perspective — is not found in these examples of public health research. We use qualitative and deconstructive strategies in research interviews and clinical examinations, but we have yet to transfer and adapt these skills and interests to other objects of study, such as audio-visual material or observational data.

Without adopting and adapting these styles of data-analysis, public health researchers restrict themselves to description and what has been called 'bean-counting', demonstrating an uncritical and unreconstructed positivism uncommon in clinical work and other areas of public health research. How, then, should the public health researcher proceed in learning about the strengths and limitations of interpretive work, so fundamental to the qualitative and deconstructive approaches?

Semiotics in public health: plain and simple

'Semiotics' is an intimidating word. It conveys complexity and mystery at the same time as sending the 'beware-of-the-dog' message — in other words, enter at your own risk. But one has to keep these things in perspective, and as with other forms of data-analysis, it is important to keep things simple, at least initially.

If someone was to introduce a person to statistical data-analysis by trying to explain multivariate analysis, this would be entirely inappropriate and intimidating. It would be ridiculous to suggest that conducting anything less than multivariate analysis is irrelevant and without merit. We know that simple descriptive statistics, even modest chi squares and T-tests, can be valuable ways of determining whether something is of interest or significance. Let us then, in the same spirit, examine some elementary principles of semiotics.

The best way to understand the study of semiotics is to remember that this is the study of interpretation — especially, but not exclusively, interpretation of language. We say 'not exclusively' because the term 'language' itself is now subject to very liberal meanings, such as the language of clothes or fashion, or 'body language'. It is valuable to remember also that the best, and most reliable, semiotics begin with a good qualitative foundation. This means that, when analysing a story or set of images, one should begin by noticing the *explicit* features, the messages deliberately being sent by the author or authors. From there, one can then move towards identification of *implicit* features.

Explicit features can be viewed as identifiable, emergent characteristics of a text, while the identification of implicit features is the result of you, as analyst, asking the text certain questions. You are prompting and probing the text for underlying features or characteristics. It is easier if you see the task in terms of different styles of enquiry.

These are the elementary questions of a qualitative analysis:
1 What is the tone of the text?
2 Note the language being used. What descriptors are being used?
3 What is the explicit aim or purpose of the story?
4 Are particular ideas or words repeated?
5 What are the major themes in the text?
6 What are the oppositional elements in the story (for example, good/bad, male/female, attachment/loss, master/servant)?

From these questions one may go on to ask more penetrating ones, looking beyond and behind the facade or appearance of the first and often taken-for-granted impressions.

We might prompt the text with some of these questions:
1 Is there a metaphor for all the separate elements or ideas in the story? Is this a 'game' perhaps? a 'rite-of-passage' perhaps? a 'morality tale'? or a 'sleight of hand'? Preposterous? Look again; look seriously for that possibility.
2 Is the story what it seemed on your first reading? Is there another way that this story might be read or interpreted? Who might read this story in this way?
3 If you have identified the explicit aims or purposes of the story, are you able to identify a less explicit agenda for the piece? What might this be?
4 Who are the 'heroes' and the 'villains' of the piece? Why are they characterised in this way?

> **5** Are there things — competing facts or ideas — that are missing from the story? If anyone else were to tell the story, would it be told in the same way or would the 'facts' be organised in roughly the same way? If not, why not?
>
> **6** Do the central ideas reflect any vested interests? What implications might this have on the story-teller's impression-management strategy — the strategy behind the words, behaviour, or visual images?

An example

It is common to examine any data with a frequency of occurrence greater than one. Sometimes the case study — a single photo, interview, or story perhaps — constitutes the basis of a study. More commonly, several episodes of behaviour or narrative are the subject of a semiotic analysis. Since we do not have room in this chapter to analyse several interviews or photographs, we have chosen to analyse a small collection of public health data for our example: all the health warnings on Australian tobacco products.

Since 1 January 1995, all cigarette packets have been required by Australian federal law to carry six health warnings. These are to be evenly and randomly distributed on all packets; they are to be written in black against a white background, must be at the front and top part of the cigarette packet, and are to be no less than 25 per cent of the total size of the space on that pack. The six messages are as follows:

SMOKING CAUSES HEART DISEASE
Government Health Warning
YOUR SMOKING CAN HARM OTHERS
Government Health Warning
SMOKING IS ADDICTIVE
Government Health Warning
SMOKING KILLS
Government Health Warning
SMOKING WHEN PREGNANT HARMS YOUR BABY
Government Health Warning
SMOKING CAUSES LUNG CANCER
Government Health Warning

The additional information to record about these warnings is that they invariably appear on cigarette packs that are gaily (sky blues, whites, reds and yellows) or stylishly (golds and silvers) coloured. They also commonly occur in conjunction with some sort of coat-of-arms emblem.

How are we to interpret these warnings as they currently appear? Let us begin with our earlier six qualitative questions.

1 Tone? The tone of the warnings is serious and authoritative. This is supported by the sober black-and-white presentation of the messages as well as the constant reminder that these are from the 'government'.

2 Language? The messages are obviously medical ('addictive', 'lung cancer', 'heart disease') and a little emotive (smoking is not said to be life-threatening; it 'kills'; a pregnant woman carries a 'baby', not a 'foetus'). They are entirely negative and threatening (smoking 'harms', 'kills', and 'causes' health problems).

3 The aim? Clearly the purposes of the messages are to discourage people from smoking, to command attention, and be taken seriously. The authors of the messages are demanding that the smoker pause to think about the messages (as demonstrated by print size, colour, and emotive language).

4 Repetition of ideas? The main idea that appears to be repeated is that of harm — to oneself and to others. Health is also another issue that is repetitive, with the messages focusing attention on the heart, lungs, and pregnancy.

5 Themes? The first theme might be described as 'self-harm'. Health is assumed to be valuable and important to everyone, and smoking threatens that health: if you value your own health, give up smoking. Four of the messages imply threats to the self. If your own health does not worry you, what about others? This is the second theme. Other people in general, and even your own children, can be harmed by smoking.

It is also worthwhile reminding readers of the use of the term 'baby' in this context. Pro-abortionists usually employ the term 'foetus', preferring a more neutral, biological descriptor than do anti-abortionists, who prefer terms such as 'child' or 'baby', which give the status of personhood to the developing foetus. We make no comment on the desirability of either, but it is useful to note that the term 'baby' has advantages over other descriptors in the additional connotations that it permits. For example, the term 'baby' can evoke ideas about family, fatherhood, motherhood, responsibility, nurture, protection, care, and so on.

6   What about possible oppositional elements? To ignore the messages implies a move away from the themes and towards its opposites: care for others versus selfishness or neglect; responsibility versus irresponsibility; health versus death and disability; seriousness versus flippancy.

The answers to our six basic questions allow us to document, with a modest degree of accuracy and fairness, the intention of those who wrote the messages. As with all qualitative work, we hope to understand, from the writers' own perspective, the central meanings important to those writers. We are also able, incidentally, to identify some of the key origins for those ideas — in this case, the medical profession and the government. But is there more to this basic description and impression of semiotics than this? Let us now make some basic semiotic moves across the data.

1   Is there a metaphor, or one main idea, that might help us draw all these separate elements and ideas together? How about the idea of 'healthism'? Crawford (1980) defines healthism as the moral style that has permeated all the central health-promotion material for many years. This is the idea that *you*, rather than anyone else, are responsible for your health.

The problem was not the design of the car, the condition of the road, or the weather; it was how *you* were driving the car that was responsible for the accident. *You* are responsible for good health. Health is within *your* control. Exercise. Exercise judgment about what and how much you should eat, drink, or smoke. Exercise physically. Exercise care on the roads, or at work. Exercise your right or the opportunity to be screened against the sun or for breast cancer. *You* are in charge, and this is serious stuff. Pay attention here.

2   You are not seriously encouraged to think about your health in any sort of political, physical, social-class, or occupational context. This may be an alternative, less explicit agenda, to be found behind the messages. Although perhaps not intentional, the possibility of this alternative interpretation suggests little or no interest in a sociological, as opposed to individualistic, view of health. Instead, the

messengers weave a morality tale that places the individual, and the individual alone, at the centre.

3 How might the messages be read in other ways? Perhaps the question should be asked in this way: How are serious messages usually read when they are presented in a wacky context? How do serious messages, purportedly from the government and doctors, look when seen on a gaily coloured box plastered with a very regal-looking coat-of-arms? How do people commonly respond on an emotional level when confronted by conflicting or paradoxical appearances? Humour? Or even just amusement perhaps? This surreal humour may help dissipate any tension caused by the initial negative emotional impact of the messages. It may also unite smokers in a context of camaraderie. Bad children laugh at their parents' dirty car as it drives down the road displaying a finger-scrawled message on the boot: 'wash me'. Everyone laughs. The multicoloured box with the coat-of-arms might just be the 'wash me' sign on every cigarette pack.

4 The 'hero' of the piece can be seen as the caring, responsible, self-controlled, family-oriented person. The 'villain' is the slovenly, dependent, and reckless person, whose habits are out of control. If these readings are possible, it is little wonder that young people are still drawn to smoking. The health warnings actually enhance their marginal self-image and encourage existing feelings of rebellion.

5 Is anything missing from the story? If health is solely *your* responsibility, several influences on health are indeed missing from these 'health warnings'. Cultural or organisational matters — such as how occupation or income determines one's access to information, health care, or safe work conditions — are ignored by or missing from 'warnings' or 'health messages'. Social psychological matters — such as how different social classes or genders think about their health and their bodies — seem to be unconsidered by the authors of the warnings. It is assumed that information is culture-neutral — that the messages do not allow different 'readings' or, if they do, that they will not be significantly different.

6 Vested interests? Clearly the messages seem to be medical in origin, and are backed by government. The term 'government' appears repeatedly with every message. Both the medical profession and governments can be seen as 'parental' figures. Is that bad? Not necessarily, but it may contribute to some people's ambivalence about that

authority. More important is the question one might ask of the abstract idea of the medical profession and government. What interest does the medical profession have in all this? Are not doctors always telling you to give something up? Why does the government take an interest in my health? Perhaps it is to save money. Then do either of those agencies *really* care about my health? Maybe, but probably no more than a mother who orders her children to eat the greens on their dinner plates; or the local council, which encourages recycling — not solely to 'save the environment' but because there is no room for rubbish tips in modern cities.

We have run out of space and time to engage in further detailed and provocative analysis using our semiotic prompts. Some of our observations might be confronting, even affronting —many semiotic interpretations are. But the following points about this exercise are worth noting.

Semiotic interpretation is a style of data-analysis aimed at exploring a variety of interpretations. It has the sociological and intellectual benefit of challenging one's own egocentrism. The way a thing appears or reads to you is not necessarily the way it may appear or read to others. Semiotic work is one way of stimulating the imagination and intellect to make way for other social and political readings (or interpretations). It is intensive case study analysis that uses some foreign prompts brought from social theories. Later, one can assess the reliability of these interpretations through the usual inter-rater means, and also assess their extent (however outrageous some of the ideas appear initially) by the usual surveys or interviews.

But however minor the extent to which an interpretation appears to be shared by people, this should not diminish its significance or importance. By identifying deeper or alternative readings as possible, and then taking them into account, health-promotion messages may be made more effective and more relevant to a wider group of people. This is an important advance in itself, and is made possible by semiotic styles of analysis. Each one of the semiotic interpretations of cigarette pack warnings has implications for the way one might construct and present the warnings in future: one could attempt to refine and control the messages being sent; or indeed, one may even reassess the wisdom of sending the message via this type of medium.

And by highlighting the social and cultural possibilities that lie in the realms of social discourse, public health semiotics shed important light on them. In this way, semiotic innovations from the humanities are capable of offering public health a novel, critical, and penetrating instrument for promoting the public good.

Some final reflections

What are some of the final lessons we might take from this brief review of models of 'good science'? Several points from our preceding discussion and arguments are worth noting. First, good science is not a technique, path, or type of thinking. Good science simply requires an imagination that can conceive of *several* styles of investigative problem solving. Sometimes something must be described carefully, fully, and sympathetically, paying attention to all the details, nuances, and complexities. Sometimes the good scholar in any science needs to be qualitative.

At other times, you will need to penetrate beneath the surface of appearances; you might need to test, experiment, cross-examine the patient, the text, or the figures before you. There are plenty of occasions when good science requires a person to stop and ask: Could the signs before me possibly mean anything other than what they appear to mean? And what are the implications associated with the answer? Sometimes, it pays to be deconstructive in one's scientific enquiries.

And, of course, there is a time to put aside description and speculation, and to anchor the theory and criticism to some careful and hopefully imaginative empirical testing. Public health research, indeed all human knowledge, is not simply a case of your interpretation against mine; it is about the way ideas and lifestyles create consequences for people.

Some of these ideas will have ambiguous political and social consequences, and arguments about their effects will be the only 'science' to test them. But many others will have measurable outcomes, quantifiable correlates, and reliable, perhaps predictable, effects, able to defeat all arguments (save those about what to do about these effects). There are times when the best, and most reformist, quality in science is its habits of measurement.

The history of public health has been a history of partnership between scientific observation and critique, beginning with protests and research into the unsanitary living conditions of the poor. This has continued right up to the present, where similar concerns are expressed in relation to the living conditions of indigenous people in Australia or the USA.

They are present in the occupational health and safety discourse around the work place, or in the design of motor vehicles. They continue in our critique of, and research into, the effects of tobacco, alcohol, or atmospheric quantities of lead.

The continuing success of these 'scientific campaigns' depends upon the effective use and adaptation of the most up-to-date methodologies and analytic strategies any academic discipline has to offer. Public health, as an interdisciplinary, modern project, has done as well as it has by drawing on the best and most useful advances in medicine and social sciences. It will continue to succeed only if it recognises that modern populations are high-tech, literary populations, and that their health is both affected and mediated by those sociological characteristics.

The deconstructive arts are one of the few contemporary methodologies able to meet the challenge that these populations now pose for the public health researcher. This is a challenge for the future of public health research, at a time when its interdisciplinary nature is being increasingly recognised as its main asset.

Recommended reading

Kaye, B. H. 1995, *Science and the Detective*, VCH Publishers, New York.

Kellehear, A. 1993, 'Unobtrusive Methods in Medical Practice Research', in General Practice Evaluation Program (ed.), *The 1993 Work-in-Progress Conference: 'Methodological Aspects of General Practice Evaluation'*, GPEP, Canberra

Kellehear, A. 1993, 'Unobtrusive Research in the Health Social Sciences', *Annual Review of Health Social Sciences*, vol. 3, pp. 46–59.

The three references above are interesting guides to unobtrusive methods in the health area.

Bayley, S. 1986, *Sex, Drink and Fast Cars*, Faber & Faber, London.

Williamson, J. 1987, *Consuming Passions*, Marion Boyers, London.

Yule, V. 1987, 'Observing Adult–Child Interaction: An Example of a Piece of Research Anyone Could Do', in M. O'Connell (ed.), *New Introductory Reader in Sociology*, Nelson, Edinburgh, pp. 69–75.

The above three references provide stimulating examples of semiotic styles of analysis in simple observations of behaviour and popular culture.

Koutroulis, G. 1990, 'The Orifice Revisited: Women in Gynaecological Texts', *Community Health Studies*, vol. 14, no. 1, pp. 73–84.

Skolbekken, J.-A. 1995, 'The Risk Epidemic in Medical Journals', *Social Science and Medicine*, vol. 40, no. 3, pp. 291–305.

The above references are some examples of the same thing, but in the health area.

Lupton, D. 1992, 'Discourse Analysis: A New Methodology for Understanding Ideologies of Health and Illness', *Australian Journal of Public Health*, vol. 16, no. 2, pp. 145–50.

A brief guide to a style of semiotic analysis.

Toulmin, S. 1990, *Cosmopolis: The Hidden Agenda of Modernity*, Free Press, New York.

And finally, an interesting and clearly written history of how our major scientific disciplines developed the methodological approaches they have today, and of why there seems to be such variance between them.

Bibliography

Aitken, P.P., Leathar, D.S., & O'Hagan, F.J. 1985, 'Children's Perceptions of Advertisements for Cigarettes', *Social Science and Medicine*, vol. 21, no. 7, pp. 785–97.

Alexander, G.R., Massey, R.M., Gibbs, T., & Altekruse, J.M. 1985, 'Firearm-Related Fatalities: An Epidemiologic Assessment of Violent Death', *American Journal of Public Health*, vol. 75, no. 2, pp. 165–8.

Anderson, I. 1996, 'Ethics and Health Research in Aboriginal Communities', in J. Daly (ed.), *Ethical Intersections: Health Research, Methods and Researcher Responsibility*, Allen & Unwin, Sydney, and Westview Press, Boulder.

Angell, M. 1990, 'The Interpretation of Epidemiological Studies', *The New England Journal of Medicine*, vol. 323, no. 12, pp. 823–5.

Anon. 1992, 'On the Future of Applied Smoking Research: Is It up in Smoke?', *American Journal of Public Health*, vol. 82, no. 1, pp. 14–16.

Armstrong, D. 1990, 'Use of the Genealogical Method in the Exploration of Chronic Illness: A Research Note', *Social Science and Medicine*, vol. 30, no. 11, pp. 1225–7.

Ashton, J. 1988, 'Tying Down the Indicators and Targets for Health for All', *Community Health Studies*, vol. 12, no. 4, pp. 376–85.

Aspinall, R.L. & Goodman, N.W. 1995, 'Denial of Effective Treatment and Poor Quality of Clinical Information in Placebo Controlled Trials of Ondansetron for Postoperative Nausea and Vomiting: A Review of Published Trials', *British Medical Journal*, vol. 311, pp. 844–6.

Astbury, J., Brown, S., Lumley, J., & Small, R. 1994, 'Birth Events, Birth Experiences and Social Differences in Postnatal Depression', *Australian Journal of Public Health*, vol. 18, pp. 176–84.

Auger, J., Kunstmann, J.M., Czyglik, F., et al. 1995, 'Decline in Semen Quality among Fertile Men in Paris During the Past 20 Years', *The New England Journal of Medicine*, vol. 332, no. 5, pp. 282–5.

Bailar, J.C. 1995, 'The Practice of Meta-analysis', *Journal of Clinical Epidemiology*, vol. 48, no. 1, pp. 149–57.

Bailey, A.J., Sargent, J.D., Goodman D.C., et al. 1994, 'Poisoned Landscapes: The Epidemiology of Environmental Lead Exposure in Massachusetts Children 1990–91', *Social Science and Medicine*, vol. 39, pp. 757–66.

Baillie, A.J., Mattick, R.P., & Hall, W. 1995, 'Quitting Smoking: Estimation by Meta-analysis of the Rate of Unaided Smoking Cessation', *Australian Journal of Public Health*, vol. 19, no. 2, pp. 129–31.

Bammer, G., Ostini, R., & Sengoz, A. 1995, 'Using Ambulance Records to Examine Nonfatal Heroin Overdoses', *Australian Journal of Public Health*, vol. 19, no. 3, pp. 316–17.

Baron, J.A., Schori, A., Crow, B., et al. 1986, 'A Randomised Controlled Trial of Low Carbohydrate and Low Fat/High Fiber Diets for Weight Loss', *American Journal of Public Health*, vol. 76, pp. 1293–6.

Barrett-Connor, E. 1979, 'Infectious and Chronic Disease Epidemiology: Separate and Unequal?', *American Journal of Epidemiology*, vol. 109, pp. 245–9.

Basch, C.E. 1987, 'Focus Group Interview: An Underutilized Research Technique for Improving Theory and Practice in Health Education', *Health Education Quarterly,* vol. 14, no. 4, pp. 411–48.

Becker, G. & Nachtigall, R.D. 1994, ' "Born to Be a Mother": The Cultural Construction of Risk in Infertility Treatment in the US', *Social Science and Medicine*, vol. 39, no. 4, pp. 507–18.

Bentham, G. 1991, 'Chernobyl Fallout and Perinatal Mortality in England and Wales', *Social Science and Medicine*, vol. 33, no. 4, pp. 429–34.

Blaze-Temple, D., Binns, C.W., & Boldy, D. 1988, 'Parental Perceptions of Measles', *Community Health Studies*, vol. 12, no. 1, pp. 55–62.

Blaze-Temple, D., Howat, P., Barney, J., et al. 1989, 'Legislative and Humanitarian Impetus for Development of Alcohol and Other Drug Policy at an Australian University', *Community Health Studies*, vol. 13, no. 4, pp. 463–70.

Bloor, M. 1976, 'Bishop Berkeley and the Adenotonsillectomy Enigma: An Exploration of the Social Construction of Medical Disposals', *Sociology*, vol. 10, no. 1, pp. 43–61.

Bloor, M. 1991, 'A Minor Office: The Variable and Socially Constructed Character of Death Certification in a Scottish City', *Journal of Health and Social Behavior*, vol. 32, pp. 273–87.

Boekeloo, B.O., Schiavo, L., Rabin, D.L., et al. 1994, 'Self-Reports of HIV Risk Factors by Patients at a Sexually Transmitted Disease Clinic: Audio vs Written Questionnaires', *American Journal of Public Health*, vol. 84, pp. 754–60.

Bonnema, J. & Dalebout, J.A. 1992, 'The Abuse of High Dose Estrogen/Progestin Combination Drugs in Delay of Menstruation: The Assumption and Practices of Doctors, Midwives and Pharmacists in a Peruvian City', *Social Science and Medicine*, vol. 34, no. 3, pp. 281–9.

Booth, T. & Booth, W. 1994, 'The Use of Depth Interviewing with Vulnerable Subjects: Lessons from a Research Study of Parents with Learning Difficulties', *Social Science and Medicine*, vol. 39, no. 3, pp. 415–24.

Bor, W., Najman, J. M., Andersen, M., et al. 1993, 'Socioeconomic Disadvantage and Child Morbidity: An Australian Longitudinal Study', *Social Science and Medicine*, vol. 36, no. 8, pp. 1053–61.

Borkan, J., Reis, S., Hermoni, D., & Biderman, A. 1995, 'Talking about the Pain: A Patient-Centered Study of Low Back Pain in Primary Care', *Social Science and Medicine*, vol. 40, no. 7, pp. 977–88.

Boutté, M.I. 1990, 'Waiting for the Family Legacy: The Experience of Being at Risk for Machado-Joseph Disease', *Social Science and Medicine*, vol. 30, no. 8, pp. 839–47.

Bowie, C., Richardson, A., & Sykes, W. 1995, 'Consulting the Public about Health Service Priorities', *British Medical Journal*, vol. 311, 28 October, pp. 1155–8.

Boyle, M.H., Torrance, G.W., Sinclair, J.C., & Horwood, S.P. 1983, 'Economic Evaluation of Neonatal Intensive Care of Very-Low-Birth-Weight Infants', *The New England Journal of Medicine*, vol. 308, June 2, pp. 1330–7.

Bremond, A., Kune, G.A., & Bahnson, C.B. 1986, 'Psychosomatic Factors in Breast Cancer Patients. Results of a Case Control Study', *Journal of Psychosomatic Obstetrics and Gynaecology*, vol. 5, pp. 127–36.

Brooks-Gunn, J., McCormick, M.C., Shapiro S., et al. 1994, 'The Effects of Early Education Intervention on Maternal Employment, Public Assistance and Health Insurance: The Infant Health and Development Program', *American Journal of Public Health*, vol. 84, pp. 924–31.

Brown, P. 1992, 'Popular Epidemiology and Toxic Waste Contamination: Lay and Professional Ways of Knowing', *Journal of Health and Social Behavior*, vol. 33, September, pp. 267–81.

Brown, S.R. 1995, 'Assessing Public Opinion on Investment in Health Services', *International Journal of Health Sciences*, vol. 6, no. 1, pp. 15–23.

Brown, S. & Lumley, J. 1993, 'Antenatal Care: A Case of the Inverse Care Law?', *Australian Journal of Public Health*, vol. 17, pp. 95–103.

Buchhorn, D. 1995, 'Food Consumption of Parents on Low Incomes', *Australian Journal of Public Health*, vol. 19, pp. 427–9.

Buck, C., Llopis, A., Najera, E., & Terris, M. 1988, *The Challenge of Epidemiology: Issues and Selected Readings*, Pan American Health Organization, Washington.

Burnstein, S., Goodhew, V., Reed, B., & Tranter, G. (eds) 1992, *Directory of Archives in Australia*, Archivists Society of Australia, Canberra.

Busschbach, J.J.V., Hessing, D.J., & De Charro, F.T. 1993, 'The Utility of Health at Different Stages in Life: A Quantitative Approach', *Social Science and Medicine*, vol. 37, pp. 153–8.

Campbell, D., Cox, D., Crum, J., et al. 1993, 'Initial Effects of the Grounding of the Tanker *Braer* on Health in Shetland', *British Medical Journal*, vol 307, 13 November, pp. 1251–5.

Campbell, L.M., Sullivan, F., & Murray, T.S. 1995, 'Videotaping of General Practice Consultations: Effect of Patient Satisfaction', *British Medical Journal*, vol. 311, 22 July, p. 236.

Cardador, M.T., Hazan, R., & Glantz, S.A. 1995, 'Tobacco Industry Smokers' Rights Publications: A Content Analysis', *American Journal of Public Health*, vol. 85, no. 9., pp. 1212–17.

Carey, V., Chapman, S., & Gaffney, D. 1994, 'Children's Lives or Garden Aesthetics? A Case Study in Public Health Advocacy', *Australian Journal of Public Health*, vol. 18, no. 1, pp. 25–32.

Carleton, R.A., Lasater, T.M., Assaf, A.R., et al. 1995, 'The Pawtucket Heart Health Program: Community Changes in Cardiovascular Risk Factors and Projected Disease Risk', *American Journal of Public Health*, vol. 85, pp. 777–85.

Carr-Hill, R. 1990, 'The Measurement of Inequities in Health: Lessons from the British Experience', *Social Science and Medicine*, vol. 31, no. 3, pp. 393–404.

Chalmers, I. & Haynes, B. 1994, 'Reporting, Updating, and Correcting Systematic Reviews of the Effects of Health Care', *British Medical Journal*, vol. 309, 1 October, pp. 862–5.

Chambless, L.E., Fuchs, F.D., Linn, S., et al. 1990, 'The Association of Corneal Arcus with Coronary Heart Disease and Cardiovascular Disease Mortality in the Lipid Research Clinics Mortality Follow up Study', *American Journal of Public Health*, vol. 80, no. 10, pp. 1200–4.

Chapman, S. 1989, 'The News on Smoking: Newspaper Coverage of Smoking and Health in Australia, 1987–88', *American Journal of Public Health*, vol. 79, no. 10, pp. 1419–21.

Chapman, S. 1993, 'Unravelling Gossamer with Boxing Gloves: Problems in Explaining the Decline in Smoking', *British Medical Journal*, vol. 307, 14 August, pp. 429–32.

Chapman, S. 1994, 'Editorial', *British Medical Journal*, vol. 309, 8 October, pp. 890–1.

Chapman, S. & Hodgson, J. 1988, 'Showers in Raincoats: Attitudinal Barriers to Condom Usage in High-Risk Heterosexuals', *Community Health Studies*, vol. 12, no. 1, pp. 97–105.

Chapman, S., Jones, Q., Bauman, A., & Palin, M. 1995, 'Incidental Depiction of Cigarettes and Smoking in Australian Magazines, 1990–1993', *Australian Journal of Public Health*, vol. 19, no. 3, pp. 313–15.

Chapman, S. & Wong, W.L. 1991, 'Incentives for Questionnaire Respondents, *Australian Journal of Public Health*, vol. 15, pp. 66–7.

Clark, P. & Bowling, A. 1990, 'Quality of Everyday Life in Long Stay Institutions for the Elderly: An Observational Study of Long Stay Hospital and Nursing Care', *Social Science and Medicine*, vol. 30, no. 11, pp. 1201–10.

Clarke, M.J. & Stewart, L.A. 1994, 'Obtaining Data from Randomised Control Trials: How Much Do We Need for Reliable and Informative Meta-analyses?', *British Medical Journal*, vol. 309, 15 October, pp. 1007–10.

Clogg, C.C. 1992, 'The Impact of Sociological Methodology on Statistical Methodology', *Statistical Science*, vol. 7, no. 2, pp. 183–207.

Cochrane, A.L. 1971, *Effectiveness and Efficiency: Random Reflections on Health Services*, The Nuffield Provincial Hospitals Trust, London.

Codlin, E. (ed.) 1990, *Directory of Information Sources in the UK*, Aslib, London.

Cole, P. 1979, 'The Evolving Case Control Study', *The Journal of Chronic Diseases*, vol. 32, pp. 15–27.

Connell, R.W., Dowsett, G.W., Rodden, P., & Davis, M.D. 1991, 'Social Class, Gay Men and AIDS Prevention', *Australian Journal of Public Health*, vol. 15, no. 3, pp. 178–89.

Conrad, P. 1990, 'Qualitative Research on Chronic Illness: A Commentary on Method and Conceptual Development', *Social Science and Medicine*, vol. 30, no. 11, pp. 1257–63.

Cook, D.J. & Guyatt, G.H. 1994, 'The Professional Meta-analyst: An Evolutionary Advantage', *Journal of Clinical Epidemiology*, vol. 47, no. 12, pp. 1327–9.

Corbett, S.J., Rubin, G.L., Curry, G.K., et al. 1993, 'The Health Effects of Swimming at Sydney Beaches', *American Journal of Public Health*, vol. 83, no. 12, pp. 1701–6.

Crawford, R. 1980, 'Healthism and the Medicalisation of Everyday Life', *International Journal of Health Services*, vol. 10, no. 3, pp. 365–89.

Crowley, S., Dunt, D., & Day, N. 1995, 'Cost-Effectiveness of Alternative Interventions for the Prevention and Treatment of Coronary Heart Disease', *Australian Journal of Public Health*, vol. 19, pp. 336–46.

Daly, E., Gray, A., Barlow, D., et al. 1993, 'Measuring the Impact of Menopausal Symptoms on Quality of Life', *British Medical Journal*, vol. 307, pp. 836–40.

Daly, J. (1997), 'Facing Change: Women Speaking about Midlife', in P. Komesaroff, P. Rothfield, & J. Daly (eds), *Reinterpreting Menopause*, Routledge, New York.

Daly, J. & McDonald, I. 1992, 'Covering your Back: Problems of Doing Qualitative Research in Clinical Settings', *Qualitative Health Research*, vol. 2, no. 4, pp. 416–38.

Danziger, S.K. 1979, 'On Doctor Watching: Fieldwork in Medical Settings', *Urban Life*, vol. 7, no. 4, pp. 513–31.

Davison, C., Frankel, S., & Smith, G.D. 1992, 'The Limits of Lifestyle: Reassessing "Fatalism" in the Popular Culture of Illness Prevention', *Social Science and Medicine*, vol. 34, no. 6, pp. 675–85.

Dawber, T.R., Kannel, W.B., & Lyell, L.P. 1963, 'An Approach to Longitudinal Studies in a Community: The Framingham Study', *Annals of the New York Academy of Sciences*, vol. 107, pp. 539–56.

Dean, K., Colomer, C., & Perez-Hoyos, S. 1995, 'Research on Lifestyles and Health: Searching for Meaning', *Social Science and Medicine*, vol. 41, no. 6, pp. 845–55.

Detels, R. 1991, 'Epidemiology: The Foundation of Public Health', in W. W. Holland, R. Detels, & G. Knox (eds), *Oxford Textbook of Public Health*, vol. 2, *Methods of Public Health*, 2nd edn, Oxford University Press, Oxford.

Dicker, A. & Armstrong, D. 1995, 'Patients' Views of Priority Setting in Health Care: An Interview Survey in One Practice', *British Medical Journal*, vol. 311, 28 October, pp. 1137–9.

Dickersin, K., Scherer, R, & Lefebve, C. 1994, 'Identifying Relevant Studies for Systematic Reviews', *British Medical Journal*, vol. 309, 12 November, pp. 1286–91.

Dodding, J. & Gaughwin, M. 1995, 'The Syringe in the Machine', *Australian Journal of Public Health*, vol. 19, no. 4, pp. 406–9.

Dodds, L., Marret, L. D., Tomkins, D.J., et al. 1993, 'Case Control Study of Congenital Anomalies in Children of Cancer Patients', *British Medical Journal*, vol. 307, 17 July, pp. 164–8.

Doll, R. & Hill, A. B. 1950, 'Smoking and Carcinoma of the Lung: Preliminary Report', *British Medical Journal*, vol. 2, 30 September, pp. 739–48.

—— 1964, 'Mortality in Relation to Smoking: Ten Years' Observations of British Doctors', *British Medical Journal*, vol. 1, pp. 1399–410 and 1460–7.

Doll, R., Peto, R., Hall, E., et al. 1994a, 'Mortality in Relation to Consumption of Alcohol: 13 Years' Observations on Male British Doctors', *British Medical Journal*, vol. 309, 8 October, pp. 911–18.

—— 1994b, 'Mortality in Relation to Smoking: 40 Years' Observations on Male British Doctors', *British Medical Journal*, vol. 309, 8 October, pp. 901–10.

Drummond, M. 1991, 'Output Measurement for Resource Allocation Decisions in Health Care', in A. McGuire, P. Fenn, & K. Mayhew (eds), *Providing Health Care: The Economics of Alternative Systems of Finance and Delivery*, Oxford University Press, Oxford, ch. 4.

Drummond, M.F., Davies, L.M., & Ferris, F.L. 1992, 'Assessing the Costs and Benefits of Medical Research: The Diabetic Retinopathy Study', *Social Science and Medicine*, vol. 34, pp. 973–81.

Drummond, M.F., Stoddart, G.L., & Torrance, G.W. 1991, *Methods for the Economic Evaluation of Health Care Programmes*, Oxford University Press, Oxford.

Dwyer, T., Coonan, W.E., Worsley, A., & Leitch, D.R. 1979, 'An Assessment of the Effects of Two Physical Activity Programmes on Coronary Heart Disease Risk Factors in Primary School Children', *Community Health Studies*, vol. 3, pp. 196–202.

Egger, M. & Smith, G.D. 1995, 'Misleading Meta-analysis', *British Medical Journal*, vol. 310, 25 March, pp. 752–4.

Elliot, H. 1995, 'Community Nutrition Education for People with Coronary Heart Disease: Who Attends?', *Australian Journal of Public Health*, vol. 19, pp. 205–10.

Elvik, R. 1995, 'The Validity of Using Health State Indexes in Measuring the Consequences of Traffic Injury for Public Health', *Social Science and Medicine*, vol. 40, pp. 1385–98.

Engels, F. 1958 (1844), *The Condition of the Working Class in England*, Basil Blackwell, Oxford.

Enkin, M., Keirse, M.J.N.C., Renfrew, M., & Neilson, J. 1995, *A Guide to Effective Care in Pregnancy and Childbirth*, Oxford University Press, Oxford.

Ennett, S.T., Tobler, N.S., Ringwalt, C.L., et al. 1994, 'How Effective is Drug Abuse Resistance Education? A Meta-analysis of Project DARE Outcome Evaluations', *American Journal of Public Health*, vol. 84, no. 9, pp. 1395–1401.

Evans, L. & Frick, M.C. 1994, 'Car Mass and Fatality Risk: Has the Relationship Changed?', *American Journal of Public Health*, vol. 84, no. 1, pp. 33–6.

Eysenck, H.J. 1994, 'Meta-analysis and its Problems', *British Medical Journal*, vol. 309, pp. 789–92.

Facione, N.C. 1993, 'Delay versus Help Seeking for Breast Cancer Symptoms: A Critical Review of the Literature on Patient and Provider Delay', *Social Science and Medicine*, vol. 36, no. 12, pp. 1521–34.

Feinstein, A. 1979, 'Methodologic Problems and Standards in Case Control Research, *Journal of Chronic Diseases*, vol. 32, pp. 35–41.

—— 1988, 'Scientific Standards in Epidemiologic Studies of the Menace of Daily Life', *Science*, vol. 242, 2 December, pp. 1257–63.

—— 1995, 'Meta-analysis: Statistical Alchemy for the 21st Century', *Journal of Clinical Epidemiology*, vol. 48, no. 1, pp. 71–9.

Feinstein, A.R., Chan, C.K., Esdaile, J.M., et al. 1989, 'Mathematical Models and Scientific Reality in Occurrence Rates for Diseases, *American Journal of Public Health*, vol. 79, no. 9, pp. 1303–4.

Fielding, N. 1993, 'Ethnography', in N. Gilbert (ed.), *Researching Social Life*, Sage, London.

Finau, S.A., Fungalei, S., Isamau, O., et al. 1986, 'Environmental and Sanitary Conditions after a Cyclone in Tonga', *Community Health Studies*, vol. 10, no. 3, pp. 336–43.

Flanders, W.D. & O'Brien, T.R. 1989, 'Inappropriate Comparisons of Incidence and Prevalence in Epidemiologic Research', *American Journal of Public Health*, vol. 79, no. 9, pp. 1301–4.

Fletcher, R.H., Fletcher, S.W., & Wagner, E.H. 1988, *Clinical Epidemiology: The Essentials*, 2nd edn, Williams & Wilkins, Baltimore.

Fook, J. 1991, 'Is Casework Dead? A Study of the Current Curriculum in Australia', *Australian Social Work*, vol. 44, no. 1, pp. 19–28.

Foucault, M. 1973, *The Birth of the Clinic: An Archaeology of Medical Perception*, Tavistock, London.

Francis, T., Napier, J.A., Voight, R.B., et al. 1955, 'Evaluation of the 1954 Field Trials of Poliomyelitis Vaccine', *American Journal of Public Health*, vol. 45, no. 5, supplement, pp. 1–63.

Frank, E., Winkleby, M., Fortmann, S.P., & Farquhar, J.W. 1993, 'Cardiovascular Disease Risk Factors: Improvements in Knowledge and Behavior in the 1980s', *American Journal of Public Health*, vol. 83, no. 4, pp. 590–3.

Franks, C. 1989, 'Preventing Petrol Sniffing in Aboriginal Communities', *Community Health Studies*, vol 13, no. 1, pp. 14–22.

French, S.A., Story, M., Downes, B., et al. 1995, 'Frequent Dieting among Adolescents: Psychosocial and Health Behaviour Correlates', *American Journal of Public Health*, vol. 85, pp. 695–701.

Gavarret, J. 1840, *Principes Généraux de Statistique Médicale*, Paris.

Geelhoed, E., Harris, A., & Prince, R. 1994, 'Cost-Effectiveness Analysis of Hormone Replacement Therapy and Lifestyle Intervention for Hip Fracture', *Australian Journal of Public Health*, vol. 18, pp. 153–60.

Gerhardt, U. 1990, 'Patient Careers in End-Stage Renal Failure', *Social Science and Medicine*, vol. 30, no. 11, pp. 1211–24.

Glaser, B. & Strauss, A. 1967, *The Discovery of Grounded Theory*, Aldine, Chicago.

Glass, G. V. 1976, 'Primary, Secondary, and Meta-analysis of Research', *Education Research*, vol. 5, pp. 3–8.

Glasziou, P.P. & Mackerras, D.E.M. 1993, 'Vitamin A Supplementation in Infectious Diseases: a Meta-analysis', *British Medical Journal*, vol. 306, 6 February, pp. 366–70.

Gliksman, M.D., Kawachi, I., Hunter, D., et al. 1995, 'Childhood Socioeconomic Status and Risk of Cardiovascular Disease in Middle Aged US Women: A Prospective Study', *Journal of Epidemiology and Community Health*, vol. 49, pp. 10–15.

Gliksman, M.D., Lazarus, R., Wilson, A., et al. 1994, 'The Western Sydney Stroke Risk in the Elderly Study: A 5-Year Prospective Study', *Annals of Epidemiology*, vol. 4, pp. 59–66.

Gliksman, M.D., Wlodarczyk, J., Heller, R.F., & Kinlay, J. 1987, 'Limitations of Telephone Based Selection and Interview Procedures', *Community Health Studies*, vol. 11, pp. 207–10.

Goodman, S.N. 1991, 'Have You Ever Meta-analysis You Didn't Like?', *Annals of Internal Medicine*, vol. 114, no. 3, pp. 244–6.

Goodman, S.N. & Royall, R. 1988, 'Evidence and Scientific Research', *American Journal of Public Health*, vol. 78, no. 12, pp. 1568–74.

Gordon, J.E. 1950, 'Epidemiology: Old and New', *Journal of the Michigan State Medical Society*, vol. 49, February, pp. 194–9.

Gorter, A., Miranda, E., Smith, G.D., et al. 1993, 'How Many People Actually Use Condoms? An Investigation of Motel Clients in Managua', *Social Science and Medicine*, vol. 36, no. 12, pp. 1645–7.

Gotay, C.C. 1991, 'Accrual to Cancer Clinical Trials: Directions from the Research Literature', *Social Science and Medicine*, vol. 33, pp. 569–77.

Grady, D., Rubin, S.M., Petitti, D.B., et al. 1992, 'Hormone Therapy to Prevent Disease and Prolong Life in Postmenopausal Women', *Annals of Internal Medicine*, vol. 117, no. 12, pp. 1016–37.

Graham, H. 1994, 'Gender and Class as Dimensions of Smoking Behaviour in Britain: Insights from a Survey of Mothers', *Social Science and Medicine*, vol. 38, no. 5, pp. 691–8.

Greenberg, M. & Schneider, D. 1994, 'Violence in American Cities: Young Black Males is the Answer, but What was the Question?', *Social Science and Medicine*, vol. 39, no. 2, pp. 179–87.

Greenland, S. 1989, 'Modelling and Variable Selection in Epidemiologic Analysis', *American Journal of Public Health*, vol. 79, no. 3, pp. 340–9.

Greenlund, K.J., Liu, K., Knox, S., et al. 1995, 'Psychosocial Work Characteristics and Cardiovascular Disease Risk Factors in Young Adults: The Cardia Study', *Social Science and Medicine*, vol. 41, no. 5, pp. 717–23.

Gregg, J. & Curry, R.H. 1994, 'Explanatory Models for Cancer among African-American Women at Two Atlanta Neighborhood Health Centers: The Implications for a Cancer Screening Program', *Social Science and Medicine*, vol. 39, no. 4, pp. 519–26.

Grund, J.-P., Kaplan, C.D., & Adriaans, N.F.P. 1991, 'Needle-Sharing in the Netherlands', *American Journal of Public Health*, vol. 81, no. 12, pp. 1602–7.

Guest, C.S., O'Dea, K., Carlin, J.B., & Larkins, R.G. 1992, 'Smoking in Aborigines and Persons of European Descent in Southeastern Australia: Prevalence and Associations with Food Habits, Body Fat Distribution and Other Cardiovascular Risk Factors', *Australian Journal of Public Health*, vol. 16, 1992, pp. 397–402.

Hall, J., Gerard, K., Salkeld, G., & Richardson, J. 1992, 'A Cost Utility Analysis of Mammography Screening in Australia', *Social Science and Medicine*, vol. 34, pp. 993–1004.

Hall, W. 1986, 'Social Class and Survival on the *S.S. Titanic*', *Social Science and Medicine*, vol. 22, no. 6, pp. 687–90.

Hall, W., Flaherty, B., & Homel, P. 1992, 'The Public Perception of the Risks and Benefits of Alcohol Consumption', *Australian Journal of Public Health*, vol. 16, no. 1, pp. 38–42.

Hallfors, D.D. & Saxe, L. 1993, 'The Dependence Potential of Short Half-Life Benzodiazepines: A Meta-analysis', *American Journal of Public Health*, vol. 83, no. 9, pp. 1300–4.

Hamid, M.A., Hussein, N.A., Bakar, A.B., & Majid, R.J.R.A. 1995, 'Cultural Beliefs and Practices during Pregnancy among Urban Squatters', *International Journal of Health Sciences*, vol. 6, no. 3, pp. 143–54.

Hammersley, M. & Atkinson, P. 1983, *Ethnography: Principles in Practice*, Tavistock, London.

Handwerker, L. 1994, 'Medical Risk: Implicating Poor Pregnant Women', *Social Science and Medicine*, vol. 38, no. 5, pp. 665–75.

Harth, S.C. & Thong, Y.H. 1995, 'Parental Perceptions and Attitudes about Informed Consent in Clinical Research Involving Children', *Social Science and Medicine*, vol. 40, pp. 1573–7.

Hassin, J. 1994, 'Living a Responsible Life: The Impact of AIDS on the Social Identity of Intravenous Drug Users', *Social Science and Medicine*, vol. 39, no. 3, pp. 391–400.

Hastings, G.B., Ryan, H., Teer, P., & MacKintosh, A.M. 1994, 'Cigarette Advertising and Children's Smoking: Why Reg was Withdrawn', *British Medical Journal*, vol. 309, 8 October, pp. 933–7.

Hatziandreu, E.I., Koplan, J.P., Weinstein, M.C., et al. 1988, 'A Cost-Effectiveness Analysis of Exercise as a Health Promotion Activity', *American Journal of Public Health*, vol. 78, 1988, pp. 1417–21.

Hazan, A.R., Lipton, H.L., & Glantz, S.A. 1994, 'Popular Films Do Not Reflect Current Tobacco Use', *American Journal of Public Health*, vol. 84, no. 6, pp. 998–1000.

Heath, C. 1986, *Body Movement and Speech in Medical Interaction*, Cambridge University Press, Cambridge.

Hedges, L.V. 1987, 'How Hard is Hard Science, How Soft is Soft Science? The Empirical Cumulativeness of Research', *American Psychologist*, vol. 42, no. 2, pp. 443–55.

Hedges, L.V. & Olkin, I. 1985, *Statistical Methods for Meta-analysis*, Academic Press, New York.

Heilbron, J. 1995, *The Rise of Social Theory*, Polity Press, Cambridge.

Helmert, U. Mielck, A. & Coassen, E. 1992, 'Social Inequities in Cardiovascular Disease: Risk Factors in East and West Germany', *Social Science and Medicine*, vol. 35, pp. 1283–92.

Helsing, K.J. & Monk, M. 1985, 'Dog and Cat Ownership among Suicides and Matched Controls', *American Journal of Public Health*, vol. 75, no. 10, pp. 1223–4.

Herman, J. 1995, 'The Demise of the Randomized Controlled Trial', *Journal of Clinical Epidemiology*, vol. 48, pp. 985–8.

Herzlich, C. & Pierret, J. 1989, 'The Construction of a Social Phenomenon: AIDS in the French Press', *Social Science and Medicine*, vol. 29, no. 11, pp. 1235–42.

Hetzel, B. 1995, 'From Papua New Guinea to the United Nations: The Prevention of Mental Defect due to Iodine Deficiency', *Australian Journal of Public Health*, vol. 19, pp. 231–4.

Heuser, L., Severson, R.K., & Watson, T.J. 1988, 'Next-of-Kin Attitudes Regarding Participation in an Epidemiologic Case-Control Study', *American Journal of Public Health*, vol. 78, no. 11, pp. 1474–6.

Higginbotham, N., Heading, G., Pont, J. et al. 1993, 'Community Worry about Heart Disease in the Coalfields and Newcastle', *Australian Journal of Public Health*, vol. 17, pp. 314–20.

Hill, A.B. 1965, 'The Environment and Disease: Association or Causation?' *Proceedings of the Royal Society of Medicine*, vol. 58, pp. 295–300.

Hill, D.J. & White, V.M. 1995, 'Australian Adult Smoking Prevalence in 1992', *Australian Journal of Public Health*, vol. 19, no. 3, pp. 305–8.

Hill, D.J., White, V.M., Borland, R., & Cockburn, J., 1991, 'Cancer-Related Beliefs and Behaviours in Australia, *Australian Journal of Public Health*, vol. 15, pp. 14–23.

Hill, D.J., White, V.M., Williams. R.M., & Gardner, G.J. 1990, 'Tobacco and Alcohol Use among Australian Secondary School Students in 1990', *Medical Journal of Australia*, vol. 152, no. 3, 15 February, pp. 124–8.

Hippocrates, 1988 'Airs, Waters, Places', in C. Buck, A. Llopis, E. Najera, & M. Terris (eds), *The Challenge of Epidemiology: Issues and Selected Readings*, Pan American Health Organization, Washington, pp. 18–19.

Hogg, R.S. 1992, 'Indigenous Mortality: Placing Australian Aboriginal Mortality within a Broader Context', *Social Science and Medicine*, vol. 35, no. 3, pp. 335–46.

Holland, W.W., Detels, R., Knox, G., et al. 1991, *Oxford Textbook of Public Health*, vol. 2, *Methods of Public Health*, 2nd edn, Oxford University Press, Oxford,

Honig, F. 1995, 'When You Can't Ask their Names: Linking Anonymous Respondents with the Hogben Number', *Australian Journal of Public Health*, vol. 19, pp. 94–6.

Houghton, S., Durkin, K., & Turbett, Y. 1995, 'Public Health Aspects of Tattooing among Australian Adults', *Australian Journal of Public Health*, vol. 19, no. 4, pp. 425–7.

Houn, F., Bober, M.A., Huerta, E.E., et al. 1995, 'The Association between Alcohol and Breast Cancer: Popular Press Coverage of Research', *American Journal of Public Health*, vol. 85, no. 8, pp. 1082–6.

Hunter. J., Schmidt, F., & Jackson, G. 1982, *Meta-analysis: Cumulating Research Findings across Studies*, Sage, Beverly Hills, Calif.

Irish, J.T. & Hall, J.A. 1995, 'Interruptive Patterns in Medical Visits: The Effects of Role, Status and Gender', *Social Science and Medicine*, vol. 41, no. 6, pp. 873–81.

Irwig, L., Cockburn, J., Turnbull, D. et al. 1991, 'Women's Perception of Screening', *Australian Journal of Public Health*, vol. 15, no. 1, pp. 24–32.

Irwin, K., Bertrand, J., Mibadumba, N., et al. 1991, 'Knowledge, Attitudes and Beliefs about HIV Infection and AIDS among Healthy Factory Workers and their Wives, Kinshasa, Zaire', *Social Science and Medicine*, vol. 32, no. 8, pp. 917–39.

Jenkins, M.A., Rubinfield, A.R., Robertson, C.F., & Bowes, G. 1992, 'Accuracy of Asthma Death Statistics in Australia', *Australian Journal of Public Health*, vol. 16, no. 4, pp. 427–9.

Jones, J. & Hunter, D. 1995, 'Consensus Methods for Medical and Health Services Research', *British Medical Journal*, vol. 311, 5 August, pp. 376–80.

Jylhä, M. 1994, 'Self-Rated Health Revisited: Exploring Survey Interview Episodes with Elderly Respondents', *Social Science and Medicine*, vol. 39, no. 7, pp. 983–90.

Kearney, M.H., Murphy, S., & Rosenbaum, M. 1994, 'Mothering on Crack Cocaine: A Grounded Theory Analysis', *Social Science and Medicine*, vol. 38, no. 2, pp. 351–61.

Kellehear, A. 1989, 'Ethics and Social Research', in J. Perry (ed.), *Doing Fieldwork: Eight Personal Accounts of Social Research*, Deakin University Press, Geelong, Vic.

—— 1990, *Dying of Cancer: The Final Year of Life*, Harwood Academic Publishers, London.

—— 1993a, 'Unobtrusive Research in the Health Social Sciences', *Annual Review of Health Social Sciences*, vol. 3, pp. 46–59.

—— 1993b, *The Unobtrusive Researcher: A Guide to Methods*, Allen & Unwin, Sydney.

King, J., Fairbrother, G., Thompson, C., & Morris, D.L. 1994, 'Influence of Socioeconomic Status, Ethnicity and an Educational Brochure on Compliance with a Postal Faecal Occult Blood Test', *Australian Journal of Public Health*, vol. 18, pp. 87–92.

Kirkman-Liff, B. & Mondragon, D. 1991, 'Language of Interview: Relevance for Research of Southwest Hispanics', *American Journal of Public Health*, vol. 81, no. 11, pp. 1399–1404.

Kitzinger, J. 1994, 'The Methodology of Focus Groups: The Importance of Interaction between Research Participants', *Sociology of Health and Illness*, vol. 16, no. 1, pp. 103–21.

Kleinman, D.L. & Cohen, L.J. 1991, 'The Decontextualisation of Mental Illness: The Portrayal of Work in Psychiatric Drug Advertisements', *Social Science and Medicine*, vol. 32, no. 8, pp. 867–74.

Kline, A., Kline, E., & Oken, E. 1992, 'Minority Women and Sexual Choice in the Age of AIDS', *Social Science and Medicine*, vol. 34, no. 4, pp. 447–57.

Knuiman, M.W., Cullen, K.J., & Bulsara, M.K. 1994, 'Mortality Trends, 1965 to 1989, in Busselton, the Site of Repeated Health Surveys and Interventions', *Australian Journal of Public Health*, vol. 18, pp. 129–35.

Knuiman, M.W., Jmrozik, K., Welborn, T.A., et al. 1995, 'Age and Secular Trends in Risk Factors for Cardiovascular Disease in Busselton', *Australian Journal of Public Health*, vol. 19, pp. 375–82.

Koestler, A. 1977, *The Act of Creation*, Picador, UK.

Konde-Lule, J.K., Musagara, M., & Musgrave, S. 1993, 'Focus Group Interviews about AIDS in Rakai District of Uganda', *Social Science and Medicine*, vol. 37, no. 5, pp. 679–84.

Kooiker, S.E. 1995, 'Exploring the Iceberg of Morbidity: A Comparison of Different Survey Methods for Assessing the Occurrence of Everyday Illness', *Social Science and Medicine*, vol. 41, pp. 317–32.

Koutroulis, G. 1990, 'The Orifice Revisited: Women in Gynaecological Texts', *Community Health Studies*, vol. 14, no. 1, pp. 73–84.

Kramer, M. 1957, 'Discussion of the Concepts of Incidence and Prevalence as Related to Epidemiologic Studies of Mental Disorders', *American Journal of Public Health*, vol. 47, pp. 826–40.

Kricker, A., McCredie, J., Elliott, J., & Forrest, J. 1986, 'Women and the Environment: A Study of Congenital Limb Anomalies', *Community Health Studies*, vol. 10, no. 1, pp. 1–11.

Krieger, N. 1992, 'The Making of Public Health Data: Paradigms, Politics and Policy', *Journal of Public Health Policy*, vol. 13, no. 4, pp. 412–27.

—— 1994, 'Epidemiology and the Web of Causation: Has Anyone Seen the Spider?', *Social Science and Medicine*, vol. 39, no. 7, pp. 887–903.

Kuh, D.J.L. & Wadsworth, M.E.J. 1993, 'Physical Health Status at 36 Years in a British National Birth Cohort', *Social Science and Medicine*, vol. 37, pp. 905–16.

La Puma, J.1992, 'Quality-Adjusted Life Years: Ethical Implications and the Oregon Plan', *Issues in Law & Medicine*, vol. 7, pp. 429–42.

Langenhoven, M.L., Rossouw, J.E., Jooste, P.L., et al. 1991, 'Change in Knowledge in a Coronary Heart Disease Risk Factor Intervention Study in Three Communities', *Social Science and Medicine*, vol. 33, pp. 71–6.

Langmuir, A. 1963, 'Surveillance of Communicable Diseases of National Importance', *The New England Journal of Medicine*, vol. 268, pp. 182–92.

Larkins, R. 1996, 'Basic Research and the Ethics of Resource Allocation', in J. Daly (ed.), *Ethical Intersections: Health research, methods and researcher responsibility*, Allen & Unwin, Sydney.

Last, J. (ed.) 1995, *A Dictionary of Epidemiology*, 3rd edn, Oxford University Press, New York.

Laurell, A.C., Noriega, M., Martinez, S., & Villegas, J. 1992, 'Participatory Research on Workers' Health', *Social Science and Medicine*, vol. 34, no. 6, pp. 603–13.

Laurence, K.M., James, N., Miller, M.H., et al. 1981, 'Double-Blind Randomised Controlled Trial of Folate Treatment before Conception to Prevent Recurrence of Neural-Tube Defects', *British Medical Journal*, vol. 282, pp. 1509–11.

Leigh, B.C., Temple, M.T., & Trocki, K.F. 1994, 'The Relationship of Alcohol Use to Sexual Activity in a US National Sample', *Social Science and Medicine*, vol. 39, pp. 1527–35.

Lerer, L.B., Butchart, A., & Terre Blanche, M. 1995, ' "A Bothersome Death": Narrative Accounts of Infant Mortality in Cape Town, South Africa', *Social Science and Medicine*, vol. 40, no. 7, pp. 945–53.

Levin, J.S. 1994, 'Religion and Health: Is There an Association, Is It Valid, and Is It Causal?', *Social Science and Medicine*, vol. 38, no. 11, pp. 1475–82.

Levy, P.S. & Lermeshow, S. 1991, *Sampling of Populations: Methods and Applications*, John Wiley & Sons, New York.

Levy, S.J. & Pierce, J.P. 1989, 'Drug Use among Sydney Teenagers in 1985 and 1986', *Community Health Studies*, vol 12, no. 2, pp. 161–9.

Lewis, S., Mason, C., & Srna, J. 1992, 'Carbon Monoxide Exposure in Blast Furnace Workers', *Australian Journal of Public Health*, vol. 16, no. 3, pp. 262–8.

Liberati, A. 1995, ' "Meta-analysis: Statistical Alchemy for the 21st Century": Discussion. A Plea for a More Balanced View of Meta-analysis and Systematic Overviews of the Effect of Health Care Interventions', *Journal of Clinical Epidemiology*, vol. 48, no. 1, pp. 81–6.

Liff, J.M., Sung, J.F.C., Chow, W-H., et al. 1991, 'Does Increased Detection Account for the Rising Incidence of Breast Cancer?', *American Journal of Public Health*, vol. 81, no. 4, pp. 462–5.

Lilienfeld, A.M. 1980, *Times, Places and Persons: Aspects of the History of Epidemiology*, Johns Hopkins, Baltimore.

Lilienfeld, A.M. & Lilienfeld, D.E. 1979, 'A Century of Case-Control Studies: Progress?', *Journal of Chronic Disease*, vol. 32, no. 5, pp. 1–13.

Link, B.G., Susser, E., Stueve, A., et al. 1994, 'Lifetime and Five-Year Prevalence of Homelessness in the United States', *American Journal of Public Health*, vol. 84, pp. 1907–12.

Lofgren, R.P., Wilt, T.J., Nichol, K.L., et al. 1993, 'The Effect of Fish Oil Supplements on Blood Pressure', *American Journal of Public Health*, vol. 83, pp. 267–9.

Loomes, G. & McKenzie, L. 1989, 'The Use of QALYs in Health Care Decision Making', *Social Science and Medicine*, vol. 28, pp. 299–308.

Louis, P.C.A. 1835, *Recherches sur les Effets de la Saignée dans quelques Maladies Inflammatoires*, Baillière, Paris.

Louis, T.A., Fineberg, H.V., & Mosteller, F. 1985, 'Findings for Public Health from Meta-analyses', *Annual Review of Public Health*, vol. 6, pp. 1–20.

Lowe, J.B., Balanda, K., Gillespie, A.M., et al. 1993, 'Sun-Related Attitudes and Beliefs among Queensland School Children: The Role of Gender and Age', *Australian Journal of Public Health*, vol. 17, no. 3, pp. 202–8.

Luepker, R.V., Jacobs Jr, D.R., Folsum, A.R., et al. 1988, 'Cardiovascular Risk Factor Change — 1973/74–80/82: The Minnesota Heart Survey', *Journal of Clinical Epidemiology*, vol. 41, pp. 825–33.

Lupton, D. 1995, 'Medical and Health Stories on the *Sydney Morning Herald*'s Front Page', *Australian Journal of Public Health*, vol. 19, no. 5, pp. 501–8.

Lupton, D. & Chapman, S. 1995, 'A Healthy Lifestyle Might be the Death of You': Discourses on Diet, Cholesterol Control and Heart Disease in the Press and among the Lay Public', *Sociology of Health and Illness*, vol. 17, no. 4, pp. 477–94.

Lupton, D., McCarthy, S., & Chapman, S. 1995, ' "Doing the Right Thing": The Symbolic Meanings and Experiences of Having an HIV Antibody Test', *Social Science and Medicine*, vol. 41, no. 2, pp. 173–80.

Macarthur, C., Foran, P.J., Bailar, J.C. 1995, 'Qualitative Assessment of Studies Included in a Meta-analysis: DES and the Risk of Pregnancy Loss', *Journal of Clinical Epidemiology*, vol. 48, no. 6, pp. 739–47.

McDonald, I.G., Daly, J., Jelinek, V.M., et al. 1996, 'Opening Pandora's Box: The Unpredictability of Reassurance by a Normal Test Result', *British Medical Journal*, vol. 313, pp. 329–32.

McGregor, O.R. 1957, 'Social Research and Social Policy in the Nineteenth Century', *The British Journal of Sociology*, vol. 8, pp. 146–57.

McIntyre, P., Hall, J., & Leeder, S. 1994, 'An Economic Analysis of Alternatives for Childhood Immunisation against Haemophilus Influenzae Type b Disease', *Australian Journal of Public Health*, vol. 18, pp. 394–400.

Mariner, W.K. 1989, 'Why Clinical Trials of AIDS Vaccines are Premature', *American Journal of Public Health*, vol. 79, pp. 86–91.

Marshall, P.A. & O'Keefe, J.P. 1995, 'Medical Students' First Person Narratives of a Patient's Story of AIDS', *Social Science and Medicine*, vol. 40, no. 1, pp. 67–76.

Mays, N. & Pope, C. 1995a, 'Observational Methods in Health Care Settings', *British Medical Journal*, vol. 311, 15 July, pp. 182–4.

—— 1995b, 'Rigour and Qualitative Research', *British Medical Journal*, vol. 311, 8 July, pp. 109–12.

Meinert, C.L. 1989, 'Meta-analysis: Science or Religion?', *Controlled Clinical Trials*, vol. 10, pp. 257S–263S.

Meyers, K., Metzger, D.S., Navaline, H., et al. 1994, 'HIV Vaccine Trials: Will Intravenous Drug Users Enroll?', *American Journal of Public Health*, vol. 84, pp. 761–6.

Mishler, E. 1984, *The Discourse of Medicine: Dialectics of Medical Interviews*, Ablex, Norwood, NJ.

Mittelmark, M.B. & Sternberg, B. 1985, 'Assessment of Salt Use at the Table: Comparison of Observed and Reported Behavior', *American Journal of Public Health*, vol. 75, no. 10, pp. 1215–16.

Montague, M. 1983, 'Baby Booms and Benefit Bludging: Are Young Women the Victims of a Myth?', *Community Health Studies*, vol. 7, no. 2, pp. 136–45.

Moore, D. 1993, 'Social Controls, Harm Minimisation and Interactive Outreach: The Public Health Implications of an Ethnography of Drug Use', *Australian Journal of Public Health*, vol. 17, no. 1, pp. 58–67.

Morgenstern, H., Glazer, W. M., Niedzwiecki, D., et al. 1987, 'The Impact of Neuroleptic Medication on Tardive Dyskinesia: A Meta-analysis of Published Studies', *American Journal of Public Health*, vol. 77, no. 6, pp. 717–24.

Morris, J.N. 1957, *Uses of Epidemiology*, Williams & Wilkins, Baltimore.

Morris, J.N., Kagan, A., Pattison, D.C. et al. 1966, 'Incidence and Prediction of Ischemic Heart Disease in London Busmen', *Lancet*, vol. 10, September, pp. 553–9.

Morris, R.D., Audet, A., Angelillo, I.F., et al. 1992, 'Chlorination, Chlorination By-products, and Cancer: A Meta-analysis', *American Journal of Public Health*, vol. 82, no. 7, pp. 955–63.

Muldoon, M.F., Maneuck, S.B., & Matthews, K.A. 1990, 'Lowering Cholesterol Concentrations and Mortality: A Quantitative Review of Primary Prevention Trials', *British Medical Journal*, vol. 301, pp. 309–14.

Mumford, E., Schlesinger, H.J., & Glass, G.V. 1982, 'The Effects of Psychological Intervention on Recovery from Surgery and Heart Attacks: An Analysis of the Literature', *American Journal of Public Health*, vol. 72, no. 2, pp. 141–51.

Najman, J. 1993, 'Health and Poverty: Past, Present and Prospects for the Future', *Social Science and Medicine*, vol. 36, no. 2, pp. 157–66.

Najman, J.M., Bor, W., Morrison, J., et al. 1992, 'Child Developmental Delay and Socioeconomic Disadvantage in Australia: A Longitudinal Study', *Social Science and Medicine*, vol. 34, no. 8, pp. 829–35.

National Health and Medical Research Council 1991, *Guidelines on Ethical Matters in Aboriginal and Torres Strait Islander Health Research*, AGPS, Canberra.

National Historical Publications and Records Commission 1988, *Directory of Archives and Manuscript Repositories in the United States*, Oryx Press, Phoenix, Ariz.

National Institutes of Health 1984, *The Use of Diagnostic Ultrasound Imaging in Pregnancy*, National Institutes of Health, Bethesda, Md.

Neave, M. 1989, 'AIDS and Women in the Sex Industry: Legal Approaches to Public Health', *Community Health Studies*, vol. 13, no. 4, pp. 423–30.

NHMRC see National Health and Medical Research Council.

Nisbet, L.A. & McQueen, D.V 1993., 'Anti-permissive Attitudes to Lifestyles Associated with AIDS', *Social Science and Medicine*, vol. 36, no. 7, pp. 893–901.

Nord, E. 1992, 'Methods for Quality Adjustment of Life Years', *Social Science and Medicine*, vol. 34, pp. 559–69.

Nord, E., Richardson, J., Street, A., et al. 1995, 'Maximising Health Benefits vs Egalitarianism: An Australian Survey of Health Issues', *Social Science and Medicine*, vol. 41, pp. 1429–37.

Oakley, A. 1985, 'Social Support in Pregnancy: The "Soft" Way to Increase Birthweight', *Social Science and Medicine*, vol. 21, no. 11, pp. 1259–68.

Oddy, W. & Stockwell, T.R. 1995, 'How Much Alcohol in Western Australia is Consumed in a Hazardous or Harmful Way?', *Australian Journal of Public Health*, vol. 19, p. 434.

Oliver, M.F. 1991, 'Might Treatment of Hypercholesterolaemia Increase Non-Cardiac Mortality?', *Lancet*, vol. 337, pp. 1529–31.

—— 1992, 'Doubts about Preventing Coronary Heart Disease: Multiple Interventions in Middle Aged Men May Do More Harm than Good', *British Medical Journal*, vol. 304, pp. 393–4.

Olkin, I. 1995, 'Statistical and Theoretical Considerations in Meta-analysis', *Journal of Clinical Epidemiology*, vol. 48, no. 1, pp. 133–46.

Olsen, J.H., Neilsen, A., & Schulgen, G. 1993, 'Residence near High Voltage Facilities and Risk of Cancer in Children', *British Medical Journal*, vol. 307, 9 October, pp. 891–9.

Opit, L. 1991, 'The Measurement of Health Service Outcomes', in W.W. Holland, R. Detels, & G. Knox (eds), *Oxford Textbook of Public Health*, vol. 2, 2nd edn, Oxford University Press, Oxford, ch. 10.

Patton, G.C., Hibbert, M., Rosier, M.J., et al. 1995, 'Patterns of Common Drug Use in Teenagers', *Australian Journal of Public Health*, vol. 19, 1995, pp. 393–9.

Patrick, D.L., Cheadle, A., Thompson, D.C. et al. 1994, 'The Validity of Self-Reported Smoking: A Review and Meta-analysis', *American Journal of Public Health*, vol. 84, no. 7, pp. 1086–93.

Peachment, A. 1984, 'Useable Knowledge and Expertise: Setting the Agenda for Tobacco Reform', *Community Health Studies*, vol. 8, no. 3, pp. 317–21.

Pierce, J.P., Yong, C.S., Dwyer, T., & Chamberlain, A. 1985, 'A Survey of Health Promotion Priorities in the Community', *Community Health Studies*, vol. 9, no. 3, pp. 263–9.

Pitts, M., Bowman, M., & McMaster, J. 1995, 'Reactions to Repeated STD Infections: Psychosocial Aspects and Gender Issues in Zimbabwe', *Social Science and Medicine*, vol. 40, no. 9, pp. 1299–1304.

Pocock, S.J., Smith, M., & Baghurst, P. 1994, 'Environmental Lead and Children's Intelligence: A Systematic Review of the Epidemiological Evidence', *British Medical Journal*, vol. 309, 5 November, pp. 1189–96.

Poole, C. 1987, 'Confidence Intervals Exclude Nothing', *American Journal of Public Health*, vol. 77, no. 4, pp. 492–3.

Quine, S. 1985 'Does the Mode Matter? A Comparison of Three Modes of Questionnaire Completion', *Community Health Studies*, vol. 9, pp. 151–6.

Rainey, D.Y. & Runyon, C.W. 1992, 'Newspapers: A Source for Injury Surveillance?', *American Journal of Public Health*, vol. 82, no. 5, pp. 745–6.

Reid, J. 1984, 'The Role of Maternal and Child Health Clinics in Education and Prevention: A Case Study from Papua New Guinea', *Social Science and Medicine*, vol. 19, no. 3, pp. 291–303.

Ridge, D.T., Plummer, D.C. & Minichiello, V. 1994, 'Knowledge and Practice of Sexual Safety in Melbourne Gay Men in the Nineties', *Australian Journal of Public Health*, vol. 18, pp. 319–25.

Riessman, C.K. 1990, 'Strategic Uses of Narratives in the Presentation of Self and Illness: A Research Note', *Social Science and Medicine*, vol. 30, no. 11, pp. 1195–200.

Rissel, C.E. 1991, 'Overweight and Television Watching', *Australian Journal of Public Health*, vol. 15, pp. 147–50.

Rissel, C.E., & Russell, C. 1993, 'Heart Disease Risk Factors in the Vietnamese Community of Southwestern Sydney', *Australian Journal of Public Health*, vol. 17, no. 1, pp. 71–3.

Roberts, M.C. & Wurtele, S.K. 1980, 'On the Noncompliant Research Subject in a Study of Medical Noncompliance', *Social Science and Medicine*, vol. 14A, p. 171.

Robinson, I. 1990, 'Personal Narratives, Social Careers and Medical Courses: Analysing Life Trajectories in Autobiographies of People with Multiple Sclerosis', *Social Science and Medicine*, vol. 30, no. 11, pp. 1173–86.

Rockett, I.R.H. & Smith, G.S. 1993, 'Covert Suicide among Elderly Japanese Females: Questioning Unintentional Drowning', *Social Science and Medicine*, vol. 36, no. 11, pp. 1467–72.

Rosendaal, F.R. 1994, 'The Emergence of a New Species: The Professional Meta-analyst', *Journal of Clinical Epidemiology*, vol. 47, no. 12, pp. 1325–6.

Ross, D.A., Kirkwood, B.R., Binka, F.N., et al. 1995, 'Child Morbidity and Mortality following Vitamin A Supplementation in Ghana: Time since Dosing, Number of Doses, and Time of Year', *American Journal of Public Health*, vol. 85, pp. 1246–51.

Ruzek, S.B. 1993, 'Towards a More Inclusive Model of Women's Health', *American Journal of Public Health*, vol. 83, no. 1, pp. 6–8.

Ryan, G.A., Barker, J.M., Wright, J.N., & McLean, A.J. 1992, 'Human Factors in Rural Road Accidents', *Australian Journal of Public Health*, vol. 16, no. 3, pp. 269–76.

Sackett, D.L. 1979, 'Bias in Analytical Research', *Journal of Chronic Diseases*, vol. 32, pp. 51–63.

Sackett, D.L. & Oxman, A.D. (eds) 1994, *The Cochrane Collaboration Handbook*, Cochrane Collaboration, Oxford.

Schacht, P.J. & Pemberton, A. 1985, 'What is Unnecessary Surgery? Who Shall Decide? Issues of Consumer Sovereignty, Conflict and Self-Regulation', *Social Science and Medicine*, vol. 20, no. 3, pp. 199–206.

Schoepf, B.G. 1993, 'AIDS Action-Research with Women in Kinshasa, Zaire', *Social Science and Medicine*, vol. 37, no. 11, pp. 1401–13.

Seamark, R. & Gaughwin, M. 1994, 'Jabs in the Dark: Injecting Equipment Found in Prisons, and the Risk of Viral Transmission', *Australian Journal of Public Health*, vol. 18, no. 1, pp. 113–16.

Seeley, J.A., Kengeya-Kayondo, J.F., & Mulder, D.W. 1992, 'Community-Based HIV/AIDS Research: Whither Community Participation? Unsolved Problems in a Research Programme in Rural Uganda', *Social Science and Medicine*, vol. 34, no. 16, pp. 1089–95.

Shiell, A. & Smith, R.D. 1993, 'A Tentative Cost-Utility Analysis of Road Safety Education', *Australian Journal of Public Health*, vol. 17, pp. 128–30.

Shyrock, R.H. 1961, 'The History of Quantification in Medical Science', in H. Woolf (ed.), *Quantification: A History of the Meaning of Measurement in the Natural and Social Sciences*, Bobbs-Merrill, Indianapolis, pp. 85–107.

Siegel, J.M., Sorenson, S.B., Golding, J.M., et al. 1989, 'Resistance to Sexual Assault: Who Resists and What Happens?', *American Journal of Public Health*, vol. 79, no. 1, pp. 27–31.

Silverman, D. 1987, *Communication and Medical Practice: Social Relations in the Clinic*, Sage, London.

Singh, G.K. & Yu, S.M. 1995, 'Infant Mortality in the United States: Trends, Differentials, and Projections, 1950 through 2010', *American Journal of Public Health*, vol. 85, no. 7, pp. 957–64.

Sirken, M.G. 1986, 'Error Effects of Survey Questionnaires on the Public's Assessments of Health Risks', *American Journal of Public Health*, vol. 76, pp. 367–8.

Skolbekken, J.-A. 1995, 'The Risk Epidemic in Medical Journals', *Social Science and Medicine*, vol. 40, no. 3, pp. 291–305.

Skrabanek, P. 1993, 'The Epidemiology of Errors', *Lancet*, vol. 342, 18 December, p. 1502.

Smith, G.D. & Phillips, A.N. 1992, 'Confounding in Epidemiological Studies: Why "Independent" Effects May Not Be What They Seem', *British Medical Journal*, vol. 305, 26 September, pp. 757–9.

Smith, G.D., Phillips, A.N., & Neaton, J.D. 1992, 'Smoking as an "Independent" Risk Factor for Suicide: Illustration of an Artifact from Observational Epidemiology?', *Lancet*, vol. 340, 19 September, pp. 709–12.

Snow, J. 1855, *On the Mode of Communication of Cholera*, John Churchill, London.

Society of Automotive Engineers 1996, *Occupant Protection Technologies for Frontal Impact: Current Needs and Expectations for the 21st Century*, SAE Publishers, New York.

Sommer, A., Tarwotjo, I., Djunaedi, E., et al. 1986, 'Impact of Vitamin A Supplementation on Childhood Mortality: A Randomised Controlled Community Trial', *Lancet*, vol. 1, pp. 1169–73.

Spitzer, W.O. 1995, 'The Challenge of Meta-analysis', *Journal of Clinical Epidemiology*, vol. 48, no. 1, pp. 1–4.

Spooner, C. & Flaherty, B. 1993, 'Comparison of Three Data Collection Methodologies for the Study of Young Illicit Drug Users', *Australian Journal of Public Health*, vol. 17, no. 3, pp. 195–202.

Stampfer, M.J., Hennekens, C.H., Manson, J.E., et al. 1993, 'A Prospective Study of Vitamin E Consumption and Risk of Coronary Disease in Women', *New England Journal of Medicine*, vol. 328, pp. 1444–9.

Steenland, N.K., Silverman, D.T., & Hornung, R.W. 1990, 'Case Control Study of Lung Cancer and Truck Driving in the Teamsters Union', *American Journal of Public Health*, vol. 80, no. 6, pp. 670–4.

Stein, H.S. & Jones, I.S. 1988, 'Crash Involvement of Large Trucks by Configuration: A Case-Control Study', *American Journal Of Public Health*, vol. 78, no. 5., pp. 491–8.

Stewart, L.A. & Parmar, M.K.B. 1993, 'Meta-analysis of the Literature or of Individual Patient Data: Is There a Difference?', *Lancet*, vol. 341, 13 February, pp. 418–22.

Stewart, W.F., Simon, D., Shechter, A., et al. 1995, 'Population Variation in Migraine Prevalence: A Meta-analysis', *Journal of Clinical Epidemiology*, vol. 48, no. 2, pp. 269–80.

Story, M. & Faulkner, P. 1990, 'The Prime Time Diet: A Content Analysis of Eating Behavior and Food Messages in Television Program Content and Commercials', *American Journal of Public Health*, vol. 80, no. 6, pp. 738–40.

Strom, B.L., Reidenberg, M.M., Freundlich, B., et al. 1994, 'Breast Silicone Implants and Risk of Systemic Lupus Erythematosus', *Journal of Clinical Epidemiology*, vol. 47, no. 10, pp. 1211–14.

Taylor, J. 1994, 'Access to Health Care for Children in Low Income Families', *Australian Journal of Public Health*, vol. 18, no. 1, pp. 111–13.

Templeton, J.F. 1987, *Focus Groups: A Guide for Marketing and Advertising Professionals*, Probus, Chicago.

Thijs, C. & Knipschild, P. 1993, 'Oral Contraceptives and the Risk of Gallbladder Disease: A Meta-analysis', *American Journal of Public Health*, vol. 83, no. 8, pp. 1113–20.

Thompson, D.C., Thompson, R.S., Rivara, F.P., et al. 1990, 'A Case Control Study of the Effectiveness of Bicycle Safety Helmets in Preventing Facial Injury', *American Journal of Public Health*, vol. 80, no. 12, pp. 1471–4.

Thompson, W.D. 1987, 'Statistical Criteria in the Interpretation of Epidemiologic Data', *American Journal of Public Health*, vol. 77, no. 2, pp. 191–4.

Threlfall, T.J. 1992, 'Sunglasses and Clothing: An Unhealthy Correlation', *Australian Journal of Public Health*, vol. 16, no. 2, pp. 192–6.

Torrance, G.W. 1976, 'Social Preferences for Health States: An Empirical Evaluation of Three Measurement Techniques', *Socio-Economic Planning Sciences*, vol. 10, pp. 29–36.

Toulmin, S. 1990, *Cosmopolis: The Hidden Agenda of Modernity*, Free Press, New York.

Towler, B., Irwig, L., Glasziou., et al. 1995, 'The Potential Benefits and Harms of Screening for Colorectal Cancer', *Australian Journal of Public Health*, vol. 19, no. 1, pp. 24–8.

Trinkoff, A.M. 1985, 'Seating Patterns on the Washington, DC Metro Rail System', *American Journal of Public Health*, vol. 75, no. 6, pp. 657–8.

Trostle, J. 1986, 'Early Work in Anthropology and Epidemiology: From Social Medicine to Germ Theory, 1840 to 1920', in C.R. James, R. Stall, & S.M. Gifford (eds), *Anthropology and Epidemiology*, D. Reidel Publishing Company, Boston.

Tsey, K. & Short, S.D. 1995, 'From Headloading to the Iron Horse: The Unequal Health Consequences of Railway Construction and Expansion in the Gold Coast, 1898–1929', *Social Science and Medicine*, vol. 40, no. 5, pp. 613–21.

Turrell, G. & Najman, J.M. 1995, 'Collecting Food-Related Data from Low Socioeconomic Groups: How Adequate are our Current Research Designs?', *Australian Journal of Public Health*, vol. 19, pp. 410–16.

Van Trigt, A.M., De Jong-Van Den Berg, L.T.W., Voogt, L.M., et al. 1995, 'Setting the Agenda: Does the Medical Literature Set the Agenda for Articles about Medicines in the Newspapers?', *Social Science and Medicine*, vol. 41, no. 6, pp. 893–9.

Vaus, D. de 1990, *Surveys in Social Research*, Unwin Hyman, London.

Venn, A., Watson, L., Lumley, J., et al. 1995, 'Breast and Ovarian Cancer Incidence after Infertility and In Vitro Fertilisation', *Lancet*, vol. 346, 14 October, pp. 995–1000.

Verhaak, P.F.M. & Tijhuis, M.A.R. 1992, 'Psychosocial Problems in Primary Care: Some Results from the Dutch National Study of Morbidity and Interventions in General Practice', *Social Science and Medicine*, vol. 35, pp. 105–10.

Victor, N. 1995, ' "The Challenge of Meta-analysis": Discussion. Indications and Contra-indications for Meta-analysis', *Journal of Clinical Epidemiology*, vol. 48, no. 1, pp. 5–8.

Viel, J.-F. & Richardson, S.T. 1993, 'Lymphoma, Multiple Myeloma and Leukaemia among French Farmers in Relation to Pesticide Exposure', *Social Science and Medicine*, vol. 37, pp. 771–7.

Viney, L.L. & Bousfield, L. 1991, 'Narrative Analysis: A Method of Psychosocial Research for AIDS-Affected People', *Social Science and Medicine*, vol. 32, no. 7, pp. 757–65.

Wachter, K.W. 1988, 'Disturbed by Meta-analysis', *Science*, vol. 241, 16 September, pp. 1407–8.

Waitzkin, H. & Britt, T. 1993, 'Processing Narratives of Self-Destructive Behavior in Routine Medical Encounters: Health Promotion, Disease Prevention and the Discourse of Health Care', *Social Science and Medicine*, vol. 36, no. 9, pp. 1121–36.

Walker, A.M. 1986, 'Reporting the Results of Epidemiologic Studies', *American Journal of Public Health*, vol. 76, no. 5, pp. 556–8.

Walker, A.M., Martin-Moreno, J.M. & Artelejo, F.R. 1988, 'Odd Man Out: A Graphical Approach to Meta-analysis', *Australian Journal of Public Health*, vol. 78, no. 8, pp. 961–6.

Walrath, J., Li, F.P., Hoar, S.K., et al. 1985, 'Causes of Death among Female Chemists', *American Journal of Public Health*, vol. 75, no. 8, pp. 883–5.

Warner, D. L. & Hatcher, R.A. 1994, 'A Meta-analysis of Condom Effectiveness in Reducing Sexually Transmitted HIV', *Social Science and Medicine*, vol. 38, no. 8, pp. 1169–70.

Warren, J.L., Bacon, E., Harris, et al. 1994, 'The Burden and Outcomes Associated with Dehydration among US Elderly, 1991', *American Journal of Public Health*, vol. 84, no. 8, pp. 1265–9.

Webb, G., Jurisich, R., & Sanson-Fisher, R. 1990, 'A Critical Review of Australian Cancer Organisations' Public Education Material', *Community Health Studies*, vol. 14, no. 2, pp. 171–9.

Weinstein, M.C. 1986, 'Risky Choices in Medical Decision Making: A Survey', *The Geneva Papers on Risk and Insurance*, vol. 11, pp. 197–216.

Weller, D.P., Owen, N., Hiller, J.E., et al. 1995, 'Colorectal Cancer and its Prevention: Prevalence of Beliefs, Attitudes, Intentions and Behaviour', *Australian Journal of Public Health*, vol. 19, pp. 19–23.

Weller, S.C. 1993, 'A Meta-analysis of Condom Effectiveness in Reducing Sexually Transmitted HIV', *Social Science and Medicine*, vol. 36, no. 12, pp. 1635–44.

Westin, S. 1990, 'The Structure of a Factory Closure: Individual Responses to Job-Loss and Unemployment in a 10-Year Follow up Study', *Social Science and Medicine*, vol. 31, no. 12, pp. 1301–11.

White, K. 1991, *Healing the Schism: Epidemiology, Medicine and the Public's Health*, Springer-Verlag, New York.

Wigglesworth, E.C. 1985, 'Occupational Accidents and Injuries: The Need for a National Data Base', *Community Health Studies*, vol. 9, no. 1, pp. 27–37.

Williams, A. 1985, 'Economics of Coronary Bypass Grafting', *British Medical Journal*, vol. 291, pp. 326–9.

Wilson, A., Bekiaris, J., Gleeson, S., et al. 1993, 'The Good Heart, Good Life Survey: Self-Reported Cardiovascular Disease Risk Factors, Health Knowledge and Attitudes among Greek-Australians in Sydney', *Australian Journal of Public Health*, vol. 17, no. 3, pp. 215–21.

Winch, P.J., Makemba, A.M., Kamazima, S.R., et al. 1994, 'Seasonal Variations in the Perceived Risk of Malaria: Implications for the Promotion of Insecticide-Impregnated Bed Nets', *Social Science and Medicine*, vol. 39, no. 1, pp. 63–75.

Winkleby, M.A., Flora, J.A., & Kraemer, H.C. 1994, 'A Community-Based Heart Disease Intervention: Predictors of Change', *American Journal of Public Health*, vol. 84, pp. 767–72.

Wolf, F. 1986, *Meta-analysis: Quantitative Methods for Research Systems*, Sage, Beverly Hills, Calif.

Wolfenden, K., McKenzie, A., & Sanson-Fisher, R.W. 1992, 'Identifying Hazards and Risk Opportunities in Child Farm Injury', *Australian Journal of Public Health*, vol. 16, no. 2, pp. 122–8.

Woodward, A., Roberts, L., & Reynolds, C. 1989, 'The Nanny State Strikes Back: The South Australian Tobacco Products Control Act Amendment Act, 1988', *Community Health Studies*, vol. 13, no. 4, pp. 403–22.

Woodward, R.V., Broom, D.H., & Legge, D. 1995, 'Diagnosis in Chronic Illness: Disabling or Enabling: The Case of Chronic Fatigue Syndrome', *Journal of the Royal Society of Medicine*, vol. 88, June, pp. 325–9.

Woolson, R.F. & Kleinman, J.C. 1989, 'Perspectives on Statistical Significance Testing', *Annual Review of Public Health*, vol. 10, pp. 423–40.

Wulff, H.R. 1976, *Rational Diagnosis and Treatment*, Blackwell Scientific Publications, Oxford.

Wyn, J. 1994, 'Young Women and Sexually Transmitted Disease: The Issues for Public Health', *Australian Journal of Public Health*, vol. 18, no. 1, pp. 32–9.

Wyn, J., Lumley, J., & Daly, J. 1996, 'Women's Health: Methods and Ethics', in J. Daly (ed.), *Ethical Intersections: Health Research, Methods and Researcher Responsibility*, Allen & Unwin, Sydney, and Westview Press, Boulder.

Yelland, J. & Gifford, S.M. 1995, 'Problems of Focus Group Methods in Cross-Cultural Research: A Case Study of Beliefs about Sudden Infant Death Syndrome', *Australian Journal of Public Health*, vol. 19, no. 3, pp. 257–63.

Index